12-2-86

Dear Stan

I hope you enjoy the book. With warm regards

[signature]

Neuropsychological
Rehabilitation
after Brain Injury

The Johns Hopkins Series in Contemporary Medicine and Public Health

Consulting Editors
Samuel H. Boyer IV, M.D.
Gareth M. Green, M.D., M.P.H.
Richard T. Johnson, M.D.
Paul R. McHugh, M.D.
Edmond A. Murphy, M.D.
Albert H. Owens, Jr., M.D.
Jerry L. Spivak, M.D.
Barbara H. Starfield, M.D., M.P.H.

Also of interest in this series:

The Perspectives of Psychiatry
Paul R. McHugh, M.D., and Phillip R. Slavney, M.D.

Practical Comprehensive Treatment of Anorexia Nervosa and Bulimia
Arnold E. Andersen, M.D.

*Family Management of Schizophrenia:
A Study of Clinical, Family, and Economic Benefits*
Ian R. H. Falloon, M.D., and Others

Neuropsychological Rehabilitation after Brain Injury

George P. Prigatano

*Head, Department of Clinical
Neuropsychology, and
Director, Neuropsychological
Rehabilitation Program,
Presbyterian Hospital,
Oklahoma City, Oklahoma*

with

David J. Fordyce
Harriet K. Zeiner
James R. Roueche
Mary Pepping
Beth Case Wood

The Johns Hopkins University Press
Baltimore and London

This book has been brought to publication with the generous assistance of
Presbyterian Hospital, Oklahoma City, and the Barrow Neurological Institute,
Phoenix, Arizona.

Dr. Prigatano is presently affiliated with the Barrow Neurological Institute,
St. Joseph's Hospital and Medical Center, Phoenix, Arizona.

© 1986 The Johns Hopkins University Press
All rights reserved
Printed in the United States of America

The Johns Hopkins University Press, 701 West 40th Street,
Baltimore, Maryland 21211
The Johns Hopkins Press Ltd, London

The paper in this book is acid-free and meets the guidelines for
permanence and durability of the Committee on Production Guidelines
for Book Longevity of the Council on Library Resources.

Library of Congress Cataloging in Publication Data

Prigatano, George P.
  Neuropsychological rehabilitation after brain injury.

  (The Johns Hopkins series in contemporary medicine and public health)
  Bibliography: p.
  Includes index.
  1. Brain damage — Patients — Rehabilitation. 2. Cognitive disorders —
Treatment. 3. Personality, Disorders of — Treatment. 4. Neuropsychology.
I. Neuropsychological Rehabilitation Program (Presbyterian Hospital, Oklahoma
City, Okla.) II. Title. III. Series. [DNLM: 1. Brain Injuries — rehabilitation.
WL 354 P951n]
RC387.5.P75   1985   616.8   85-8061
ISBN 0-8018-2644-6 (alk. paper)

To the Memory of
Kurt Goldstein

> *More than any other modern clinician, he was able to capture in words the plight of brain-injured patients.*

Contents

Contributors	xiii
Foreword, by Sheldon Berrol, M.D.	xv
Preface	xvii
Introduction	xix

1. Cognitive Dysfunction and Psychosocial Adjustment after Brain Injury   1
    George P. Prigatano and David J. Fordyce
    The Problem of Defining Cognition and Cognitive Dysfunction   3
    Common Cognitive Dysfunctions and Their Psychosocial Outcomes   4
    Unrealistic Self-appraisal after Brain Injury   12
    The Problem of Unemployment   14
    Summary   16

2. Nonaphasic Language Disturbances after Brain Injury   18
    George P. Prigatano, James R. Roueche, and David J. Fordyce
    The Problem of Talkativeness   20
    The Problem of Tangentiality   21
    The Phenomenon of Peculiar Phraseology   23
    Summary   27

3. Personality and Psychosocial Consequences of Brain Injury   29
    George P. Prigatano
    Neuropsychological Considerations of Personality   30
    Common Personality Disturbances after Brain Injury   33
    Personality Disturbances in Brain-injured Children   43
    A Schema for Classifying Personality Disorders   44

Psychosocial Consequences   46
Summary   49

4. Cognitive Retraining in Perspective   51
   George P. Prigatano
   The Historical Perspective   52
   The Clinical Perspective   56
   The Research Perspective   64
   Summary   66

5. Psychotherapy after Brain Injury   67
   George P. Prigatano
   Goals of Psychotherapy after Brain Injury   69
   Elements of Psychotherapeutic Intervention   71
   A Schema for Conducting Psychotherapy after Brain Injury   74
   Individual Psychotherapy   74
   Group Psychotherapy   77
   The Importance of Symbolism in the Therapeutic Process   83
   Predictable Psychotherapeutic Problems   88
   Education, Social Support, and Psychotherapy of
       Family Members   92
   The Reactions of Professional Staff to Brain-injured Patients   94
   Summary   95

6. The Neuropsychological Rehabilitation Program at
   Presbyterian Hospital, Oklahoma City   96
   George P. Prigatano and David J. Fordyce
   Philosophy and Rationale   98
   Selection of Patients   100
   The Program   102
   Medical Consultants   114
   Staff Development and Interdisciplinary Staff Relationships   114
   Initial Impressions and Ideas Concerning Outcome Measures   115
   Summary   118

7. The Outcome of Neuropsychological Rehabilitation Efforts   119
   George P. Prigatano, David J. Fordyce, Harriet K. Zeiner,
   James R. Roueche, Mary Pepping, and Beth Case Wood
   Subjects   120
   Neuropsychological Tests   122
   Personality Tests   122
   The Follow-up Interview   124
   Analysis and Findings of the Neuropsychological Tests   124
   Personality Test Findings   127
   Work Status during Follow-up   128

The Effectiveness of Neuropsychological Rehabilitation 130
Summary 132

8. Modification of the Neuropsychological Rehabilitation Program at Presbyterian Hospital, Oklahoma City 134
   George P. Prigatano
   The Modified Program 134
   Clinical Observations 135

Appendix A. Patient Competency Rating (Patient's Form), Neuropsychological Rehabilitation Program, Presbyterian Hospital 143

Appendix B. Patient Competency Rating (Relative's Form), Neuropsychological Rehabilitation Program, Presbyterian Hospital 147

Appendix C. Revisions to the Neuropsychological Rehabilitation Program at Presbyterian Hospital 152

References 165

Author Index 175

Subject Index 179

Figures

1.1. Lateral View of the Left Cerebral Hemisphere and Common Areas of Contusion Associated with Severe Craniocerebral Trauma 2
2.1. Reportedly Normal CT Scan in a Young Adult Female Patient with Significant Neuropsychological Sequelae after Severe Craniocerebral Trauma 24
2.2. EEG Recording in the Same Patient Several Months Postinjury 25
3.1. Galvanic Skin Response to Emotional and Nonemotional Stimuli in Patients with Dominant and Nondominant Hemispheric Lesions 39
4.1. CT Scan Demonstrating Bilateral Frontal Atrophy in a Young Adult Male after Severe Craniocerebral Trauma 58
4.2. Cerebral Angiogram Revealing an Arteriovenous Malformation Involving the Corpus Callosum in a Young Adult Male before Surgical Removal 60
5.1. Common Misperceptions of What Occurs in Psychotherapy 75
5.2. Spontaneous Drawing by a Young Adult Brain-injured Patient *facing 84*
5.3. A Second Drawing from the Same Patient *facing 85*

5.4. Spontaneous Drawing by a Traumatic Head-Injury Patient at the Completion of a Rehabilitation Program   85
5.5. Drawing by an Adolescent Head-injured Boy   86
5.6. A Second Drawing from the Same Patient   87
7.1. Scores on Intelligence and Memory Tests of NRP Patients and Control Subjects   128

Tables

1.1. Ischemic Brain Damage Associated with Severe Craniocerebral Trauma   9
2.1. Katz-Relatives' Form Ratings of 48 Brain-injured Patients Classified as "Talkative" or "Not Talkative"   21
3.1. Model for Assessing Psychosocial Outcome after Brain Injury   47
7.1. Demographic and Neurological Characteristics of NRP Patients   121
7.2. Demographic and Neurological Characteristics of Control Subjects   123
7.3. Average Wechsler Test Scores of NRP Patients and Control Subjects before and after Treatment   126
7.4. Average Neuropsychological Test Scores of NRP Patients and Control Subjects before and after Treatment   127
7.5. Katz Adjustment Scale Z Scores of NRP Patients and Control Subjects before and after Treatment   129
8.1. Demographic and Neurological Characteristics of 40 Patients Completing the NRP (February 1980 to February 1984)   136
8.2. Mean Neuropsychological Test Scores of NRP Patients   137
8.3. Mean Katz-R Test Scores of NRP Patients   138
8.4. Duncan Multiple-range Scores on Katz-R Data for NRP Patients   139

Contributors

DAVID J. FORDYCE, Ph.D., past co-director, Neuropsychological Rehabilitation Program, Presbyterian Hospital, Oklahoma City, Oklahoma

MARY PEPPING, Ph.D., present co-director, Neuropsychological Rehabilitation Program, Presbyterian Hospital, Oklahoma City, Oklahoma

GEORGE P. PRIGATANO, Ph.D., Head, Department of Clinical Neuropsychology, and Director, Neuropsychological Rehabilitation Program, Presbyterian Hospital, Oklahoma City, Oklahoma

JAMES R. ROUECHE, M.S., speech and language pathologist, Neuropsychological Rehabilitation Program, Presbyterian Hospital, Oklahoma City, Oklahoma

BETH CASE WOOD, O.T.R., occupational therapist, Neuropsychological Rehabilitation Program, Presbyterian Hospital, Oklahoma City, Oklahoma

HARRIET K. ZEINER, Ph.D., research psychologist, Neuropsychological Rehabilitation Program, Presbyterian Hospital, Oklahoma City, Oklahoma

Foreword

Functional recovery after brain damage has been debated in the literature for many years. The old concept of the central nervous system as a static, all-or-none unit has gradually eroded as clinicians involved in rehabilitation have outlined substantial functional change over time. The incorporation of behavioral theory and learning theory in the remediation process has gradually expanded our potential to direct change beyond that incurred by the physical level of disability. The program at Presbyterian Hospital in Oklahoma City, which is the basis for this volume, represents a highly structured system of interventions that clearly demonstrates the potential for positive behavioral change, providing the brain-damaged individual with a broader array of coping strategies and deficit remediation. The focus of the program is dealing with a deficit as it impinges on a social behavior, thus providing the basis for ultimate reintegration into the community. Thus, we see that Dr. Prigatano approaches not only the cognitive disturbances but also the personality and behavioral consequences of brain disruption that are all too frequently neglected in traditional rehabilitation programs.

Failures in traditional rehabilitation are commonly said to be a result of motivational problems. Outlined in this volume is a hierarchical approach to reestablishing basic goal-seeking behaviors that form the foundation of motivation. Unless rehabilitation efforts are directed at disturbances of attention, concentration, and information-processing, one cannot hope to achieve realistic motivational capacity.

A major emphasis of the program is directed toward helping the family deal not only with the altered individual who results from brain injury but also with the altered social structure that results within the family unit and as the family relates to the community. It has long been recognized that an intact, functioning social unit is essential to the maintenance of long-range rehabilitation goals. Thus, the recognition of family needs and the establishment of an adequate support system to meet the ongoing needs of the family as well as of the patient remain fundamental components of an effective rehabilitation program.

Cognitive remediation is a relatively new term that has become fashionable in the rehabilitation community, but the basic concepts of cognitive retraining have been established and widely accepted in the special education community for years. However, cognitive retraining that does not deal with goal-directed behaviors, personality deficits, and behavioral consequences is just another fragmented, isolated approach. A developmental structure in a balanced program that allows sufficient flexibility in utilizing compensation training, substitution training, and specific deficit remediation dependent on the functional abilities of the individual appears to have greater rewards for the rehabilitation process.

Dr. Prigatano's program has demonstrated that incorporation of a therapeutic community environment results in substantial improvement in functioning, but he almost apologizes for the modest improvement in standardized neuropsychological testing. It may well be that standardized neuropsychological testing does not always correlate well with functional outcomes. The hallmark of this program, however, is that patients demonstrate more organized behavior, a lower level of confusion, a significant increase in interpersonal skills, and a significant decrease in emotional stress. Thus, an individual going through such a program becomes more functional within the community and in the society in general.

We now know that recovery can occur in the brain-damaged individual. The question that has long been facing the rehabilitation community is what can be done to maximize the degree of recovery. The program at Presbyterian Hospital has taken a major step forward in exposing this potential.

Sheldon Berrol, M.D.
Chief, Rehabilitation Medicine Services
San Francisco General Hospital
San Francisco, California

Preface

The Neuropsychological Rehabilitation Program at Presbyterian Hospital in Oklahoma City has been in existence for more than five years. During this time the program staff have worked intensively with a number of patients to help them cope with their brain injuries and reconstruct a productive life-style. In the course of this work, various papers were written (many of which are cited in this volume) to define the nature of the higher cerebral deficits associated with brain injury, particularly traumatic closed head injury. Because the emphasis of the program was on helping these patients return to some semblance of normal living, it was inevitable that our description of the cognitive and personality deficits would be couched in terms of their impact on psychosocial adjustment. Also, attempts of neuropsychologically oriented intervention were aimed not at improving a specific deficit in isolation but at dealing with that deficit as it impinged on a broader class of social behaviors.

We began this venture specifically concerned with the relationship between the brain and behavior, but it became obvious that a broader perspective was needed in order to work with the patients successfully. As the chapters in this volume reflect, ideas that have been useful to us have come from clinical psychology, psychiatry, neurology, neurosurgery, neuropsychology, and psychoanalysis. Without a broad clinical perspective, it would be impossible to deal with the multitude of problems experienced by brain-injured patients, their families, and the rehabilitation staff who attempt to help them. It is hoped that this volume will prove useful to those who wish to help brain-injured patients reestablish a sense of productivity, and therefore meaning, in their life.

Presbyterian Hospital was the prime mover in supporting this work. Hospital administrators gave free rein to the neuropsychology staff in developing the various ideas and therapeutic procedures. Proceeds obtained by distributing this volume will be returned to the hospital to further research in the rehabilitation of brain-injured patients. Special thanks are extended to Harry Neer, President of Presbyterian Hospital, and Barton Carl, M.D., Chief of Neurosurgery. More than any other individuals, their support made the program a reality. Also, the administrative support of Dennis Millirons, Vice President of Operations and Professional Departments, is happily recognized. While concerned with the financial feasibility of our program, President Neer and Vice President Millirons never limited our growth on the basis of purely fiscal issues. Few clinical directors can boast of such faith and support in a department's activities. Finally, the work of numerous secretaries should be recognized in preparing this book and helping run our day-to-day clinical and research activities; Ardith Davis, Virginia Hodam, and Executive Secretary Linda Modisette deserve special recognition.

Introduction

Craniocerebral trauma produces alterations at various levels of brain function. These changes are difficult to understand scientifically, but their clinical manifestations are quite predictable. Changes in cognitive functioning, as well as disorders of personality, occur frequently. The result is a major problem of psychosocial adjustment for the patient and his or her family.

Because of the position in which the human brain sits within the skull, traditional views of the neuropathology of closed-head injury have emphasized the vulnerability of the tips of the frontal lobe, the tips of the temporal lobe, and brain-stem structures (Russell 1971; Levin, Benton, and Grossman 1982). However, research has emphasized that there are many types of "brain damage" associated with craniocerebral trauma. In addition to the shearing effects, one can see areas of hemorrhage as well as ischemic damage. Basal ganglia and hippocampal structures may be especially susceptible to the latter form of injury (Graham, Adams, and Doyle 1978). Thus, brain-damaged patients frequently have problems of memory, emotion, and motivation that appear to have a clear organic basis. Impulsivity, irritability, paranoid ideation, and impaired judgment also seem to be mediated in part by the myriad of neurological lesions common in these patients.

Until recently, these observations discouraged many people from attempting cognitive remediation or skills-retraining with brain-injured patients. There is also still considerable resistance to attempting psychotherapy with brain-injured patients, since it is assumed that they will not benefit from such intervention. Yet the degree of brain injury is quite variable from patient to patient, and patients' premorbid cognitive and personality characteristics are not uniform. Having suffered brain injury, these individuals are confused and have predictable fragmented feelings of depression, anger, and hopelessness. They search for some understanding of what has happened to them and, like everyone else, attempt to reestablish meaning in their life after a major personal tragedy.

The primary aim of this volume is to describe the long-term cognitive and personality disturbances that are seen after severe traumatic brain injury. It makes the argument that both cognitive remediation and psychotherapy should be attempted after brain injury, and comprehensive neuropsychological rehabilitation includes both activities. In addition to working with the patients directly, family members and even the professional staff that care for the patients require educational and interpersonal support to facilitate the rehabilitation outcome. Families can become discouraged, irritated, and hopeless, and staff committed to the patients' care experience the same emotional reactions. Consequently, in attempting rehabilitation, one must take a broad perspective on the possible causes of behavioral disturbance in the patients, family, and staff. This involves integrating ideas not only from neuropsychology but also from clinical psychology, psychiatry, and psychoanalysis. With a truly clinical approach, one can define the major variables that get in the way of patients' learning to make reasonable commitments in life. Staff members also need assistance in dealing with the confusion such patients inevitably generate.

This volume is the outgrowth of experiences in working with brain-injured patients. Chapters 1, 2, and 3 deal with the cognitive, linguistic, and personality disturbances frequently associated with traumatic head injury, disturbances that persist in some form several months and even years after the injury. In fact, total recovery seldom occurs after significant brain injury. The book also focuses on what is meant by cognitive retraining and psychotherapy after brain injury. Chapters 4 and 5 are primarily for rehabilitation specialists struggling with developing a framework for approaching the cognitive and personality problems seen in brain dysfunctional patients.

Chapter 6 describes the Neuropsychological Rehabilitation Program at Presbyterian Hospital in Oklahoma City, and Chapter 7 presents the outcome of the program's initial clinical efforts. Chapter 7 also makes it clear that there is a need to expand therapeutic activities to include a protected or at least closely supervised work trial. Chapter 8 summarizes the state of evolution the program has gone through (the revised program is described in Appendix C) and includes clinical impressions and psychometric data on a larger group of forty patients seen during the first four years of the program. The patients were described as successes, failures, and intermediates, and their neuropsychological and personality characteristics are described in some detail. These groups included not only traumatically head-injured patients but also a few patients with localized nontraumatic lesions.

The material presented here helps clarify what chronically brain-injured young adults experience several months or years postinjury and provides guidelines for their clinical management and eventual rehabilitation. These patients are frequently not adequately assessed or treated because their disturbances in higher cerebral functioning are poorly understood. In addition, they tend to eventually alienate family, friends, and even rehabilitation staff, and as a result may be discharged from rehabilitative care because people do not know how to treat them or want to treat them in view of their social impact on others. Only by a combination of scientific insight and sensible clinical care can these patients and their families hope to reestablish some sense of productivity and meaning in their lives.

Neuropsychological
Rehabilitation
after Brain Injury

CHAPTER 1
Cognitive Dysfunction and Psychosocial Adjustment after Brain Injury

George P. Prigatano and David J. Fordyce

Craniocerebral trauma in young adulthood produces predictable alterations in cognitive functioning. Some cognitive impairments improve with time, others are resistant to change but may slowly improve with time and treatment, still others are relatively permanent. The severity of the brain injury and the areas of cortical and subcortical damage are the two major predictors of residual cognitive dysfunction.

The severity of the injury, as reflected by measures of duration of coma or posttraumatic amnesia, has been related in studies to the degree of neuropsychological impairment, employment status, and alterations in personality (e.g., Levin et al. 1979; Rimel et al. 1981, 1982). These studies, however, typically report on scores taken from neuropsychological tests and do not specify the underlying nature of the residual cognitive deficits except in very broad terms. Consequently, the identification of areas of cognitive dysfunction that substantially interfere with the patient's psychosocial adjustment generally has come from working with patients in the rehabilitation setting (see Goldstein 1942). While this is a limited approach, it is the best available at present.

Relating areas of brain dysfunction to residual cognitive disturbances has been difficult because this patient group is quite heterogeneous in terms of the nature and severity of its neuropathology. Adams (1975) pointed out that no two head-injured patients are alike because of this neuropathological phenomenon. The neuropathological insults associated with brain injury are both primary and secondary in nature; that is, there is direct structural damage due to shearing of white matter as well as secondary damage associated with such processes as hypoxia and hematomas. While certain brain regions are at high risk for injury, virtually all areas of the brain can be damaged. Clinically, one frequently finds neurobehavioral evidence indicative of anterior frontal lobe and anterior temporal lobe injury (see Fig. 1.1), and brain-stem injury (Ommaya and Gennarelli 1974).

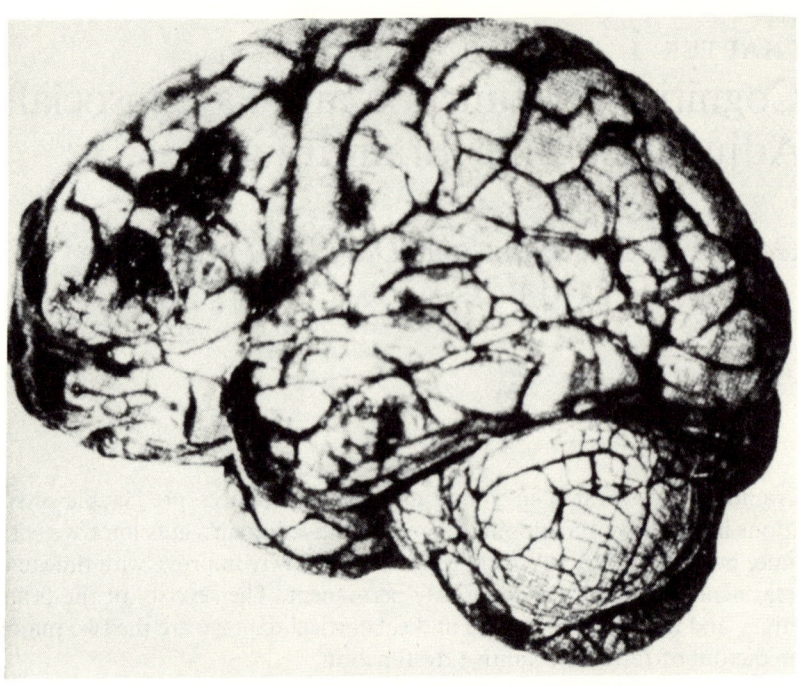

Figure 1.1. Lateral View of the Left Cerebral Hemisphere and Common Areas of Contusion Associated with Severe Craniocerebral Trauma. Reprinted, by permission, from W. R. Russell, *The Traumatic Amnesias* (London: Oxford University Press, 1971).

Many, if not all, patients with severe head injury show disturbances that suggest that these regional areas have been compromised in their functional integrity (Levin et al. 1982). Typically, these patients are impulsive, have poor judgment, misperceive the intentions or actions of others, are slow in processing information, and complain of memory disturbance. Sleep studies have also suggested possible underlying neurophysiological disturbances that may contribute to these neurobehavioral problems (see Prigatano et al. 1982).

Severe head injury is defined as an injury causing a patient to have Glasgow Coma Scale (GCS) scores between 3 and 8 and/or a period of unconsciousness greater than twenty-four hours. The disturbances that will be described have been identified as a result of working with patients intensively in the Neuropsychological Rehabilitation Program (NRP) at Presbyterian Hospital in Oklahoma City (the program is outlined in detail in Chapter 6). Since this patient group was worked with from the perspective of trying to get the patient back to gainful employment and improving interpersonal adjustment, the relationship between various cognitive dysfunctions and psychosocial adjustment was under constant clinical scrutiny. This chapter relates cognitive disturbances to the psychosocial outcome. Research that appears to be relevant to these clinical problems, as encountered by the rehabilitation-oriented psychologist, will also be discussed. The reader is referred to other sources for a more comprehensive view of the research that deals with cognitive disturbance after traumatic brain injury (see Levin et al. 1982; Newcombe and Ratcliff 1979).

The Problem of Defining Cognition and Cognitive Dysfunction

A perplexing problem in the neurosciences has been the question "How does the brain code information?" Pribram (1977) argued for holographic principles. Hubel and Wiesel emphasized the feature-detection characteristics of simple and complex cells (see Kuffler and Nicholls 1977). Neurophysiological and neurochemical analyses of brain function abound, but the basic mystery remains (Eccles 1977). Neuropsychological and computerized information-processing models of brain function add more complexities to this basic question. Luria (1966) pointed out that the activities of brain function are clearly interrelated. The higher cerebral or mental functions (of which the term *cognition* certainly in part applies) seem to emerge as a result of several functional subsystems working together. These mental functions are also social in origin, according to Luria (1966). That is, contact of the developing child (nervous system) with a given environment determines to a large extent how a child interprets or perceives information. Finally, the work of Simon (1967) emphasized that no theory of thinking (or cognition) is complete without integrating the concepts of emotion and motivation. Thinking or problem-solving does not occur in a vacuum. Feelings about a given problem or solution have a profound impact on how we think. They guide us to pursue a topic or abandon it despite the "logical" evidence for one or the other.

These considerations led to the conclusions that there is no simple definition of the word *cognition* (Flavell 1977) and that cognition or cognitive deficits cannot be defined devoid of the concepts of emotion and motivation (Simon 1967). Yet to help identify the higher cerebral deficits of brain-injured patients, it may be useful to focus on specific types of information-processing deficits and how they relate to the patient's ability to cope in society.

The term *cognition* will be used to refer to the basic ability of the brain to process, store, retrieve, and manipulate information to solve problems. Information presented to the brain-injured patient by psychologists in a rehabilitation setting typically involves formal psychological testing, structured interviews, and performance on standardized sensory and motor tasks. Thus, much of the research on the relationship of cognitive deficit to psychosocial outcome focuses on the relationship of test scores to broad categories of social adaptation. Within the confines of the NRP at Presbyterian Hospital, however, brain-injured patients are worked with from a traditional neuropsychological test point of view and are also seen in a series of cognitive and psychotherapeutic activities. They are worked with individually, in small-group activities, and in a therapeutic environment. These various activities have allowed a broader sample of their behaviors and perhaps a more representative indication of how they would function in nonrehabilitative settings. In addition, their families are worked with on a weekly basis so we can develop a list of cognitive deficits that appear to have great impact on the patient's ability to adjust in both the work environment and the home environment.

Common Cognitive Dysfunctions and Their Psychosocial Outcomes

The cognitive disturbances encountered with traumatic brain-injured patients are as follows:

Disorders of Attention and Concentration

Trouble sustaining attention; easy fatigability
Impaired selective attention and scanning
Poor shifting of attention back and forth, so the patient frequently "gets lost" in group communication

Disorders of Initiation and Planning of Goal-Directed Activities

Impairment of the abstract attitude; patient frequently missing the point and taking information literally, not symbolically
Trouble inhibiting action before action is required or after it should stop, resulting in impulsive and perseverative responses
Slowness in initiation time
Confusion as to where to start in solving a problem and consequently often using unrealistic problem-solving strategies
Difficulty ordering or sequencing information
Difficulty knowing when, where, and how to ask for help
Trouble learning from mistakes as well as from successes

Disorders of Judgment and Perception

Misinterpretation of actions or intentions of others
Confusion on being presented with multiple bits of information at one time
Tendency to be socially inappropriate in verbal communications
Unrealistic appraisal of self and residual strengths and weaknesses after brain injury.

Disorders of Learning and Memory

Poor rote learning

Material-specific short-term memory deficits (e.g., verbal versus nonverbal)
Difficulty organizing or processing information that is "important to remember," particularly as it relates to academic or work skills
Amnestic disturbance (in some patients) (i.e., Memory Quotient substantially below IQ)

Disorders of the Speed of Information-Processing
Extreme slowness in reaction time
Slowness in psychomotor activities (e.g., talking, writing, doing mechanical tasks)

Disorders of Communication (Aphasic and Nonaphasic)
Anomia
Inefficient word retrieval
Tangentiality of thought and speech
Talkativeness
Use of peculiar words and phrases
Uninhibited choice of words (i.e., four-letter superlatives)

To varying degrees, these disturbances exist in most, if not all, traumatically brain-injured young adults. The pattern of deficits and their severity depend on the neuropathological insults.

DISORDERS OF ATTENTION AND CONCENTRATION

Complaints of easy fatigability, increased need for sleep, and poor attentional skills are common in head-injured patients. Van Zomeren (1981) reported this and, using a reaction-time paradigm, studied attentional disturbances and their recovery over time. His work demonstrates that the degree of attentional deficit is related to the severity of the brain injury. Moreover, the time course for recovery may exceed two years postinjury. Choice reaction time seems to be especially predictive of eventual neurological and social outcome (Van Zomeren and Deelman, 1978). Choice reaction time scores at five months postinjury correlated with the Glasgow Outcome Scale ($r = +.72$) at twelve months postinjury. The faster times were clearly associated with better overall neurological recovery. Social outcome (as measured by a composite score for work status, family life and leisure activity) was also related to this reaction-time measure ($r = +.48$).

The attentional deficits of traumatically brain-injured patients can be obvious or subtle. When these patients are actively engaged by an examiner or therapist, their attentional skills may appear to be adequate. This is because the environment is now structured and provocative. However, if such patients are left on their own to attend to information, the deficits often become more pronounced. The internal regulatory system (or systems) that help shift and maintain attention are faulty. Fuster's (1980) description of attentional disorders manifested by easy distractibility and difficulty maintaining concentration following prefrontal cortical ablations in monkeys was strikingly similar to what one sees in the clinical setting with brain-injured patients.

Attentional disturbances of traumatically brain-injured individuals are also evidenced in a social interaction when many people are working and talking together in a group. If the patient is directly engaged by a given individual in the context of the conversation, attentional skills appear to be within normal limits; but if more than one person is talking, or if the topic of conversation is not particularly relevant to his or her perceived needs, the patient becomes easily distractible and may engage in tangential comments. Many of these patients are often not aware of their tangentiality, even though they can identify their attentional disturbance. This often leaves others with the impression that the brain-injured patient is egocentric, selfish, or perhaps experiencing major psychiatric disturbances because of his or her uninhibited and distractible nature. Employers cannot tolerate this type of behavior, and old friendships quickly dissolve in the face of it. As a consequence, focusing on remediation of or compensation for attentional deficits, particularly in unstructured group activities, is vital for an ultimate rehabilitation success with these patients. Ben-Yishay et al. (1982) have recognized this for some time and have tried to develop a series of training "modules" to deal with these attentional disturbances. While these disturbances are also informally dealt with in the context of group work through Ben-Yishay's program, the technology for dealing with attentional disturbances in interpersonal interaction has been underdeveloped.

DISORDERS OF INITIATION AND PLANNING OF GOAL-DIRECTED ACTIVITIES

A common complaint of relatives of significantly impaired brain-injured young adults after they return home from traditional rehabilitation is that they frequently show a lack of initiative and have to be told what to do. This can be misinterpreted as primarily a psychiatric problem, but many such patients simply lack the cognitive skills to know how and when to carry out various goal-directed activities. Prior to their injury, they may have been able, for example, to take care of household chores spontaneously as those chores became obvious to them; but now these patients may sit and wait to do the chores until specifically told to do so. On formal testing, these patients show clear disturbances in abstract reasoning. They also seem to demonstrate what Luria (1966) referred to as a disorder in the kinetics of motor planning, which is frequently seen with prefrontal injuries. Each motor act seems to be disconnected or disjointed and is not carried out in a smooth, interconnected fashion, so the flow of goal-directed activity is easily disrupted. The patient often remains in a state of psychological inertia because the cognitive steps or "programming" necessary to carry out complex action are simply not present or are greatly impaired. Usually these patients will do what they are told without any objection and in a very literal manner when instructions come from the environment. This type of reaction can be separated from psychiatrically based inertia. When the latter occurs, the patient is often irritated or belligerent when given specific instructions to carry out activities. It is important to separate these two types of phenomena when working with brain-injured patients.

In its severe form, this type of initiation and planning disorder can be accompanied by pronounced perseverative errors. Once engaging in an activity, the patient may find it difficult to inhibit or stop that activity. Neuropsychologists frequently see this phenomenon on such tests as the Wechsler Memory Scale, in which the individual is asked to draw Design 2, which includes producing sixteen dots. Once dot-making begins, the patient may persist and produce three or four times the number of dots needed.

While this type of disturbance is certainly obvious when it occurs in its severe forms, it may exert important but subtle effects on the moderately impaired brain-injured patient. For example, executives who have suffered mild or moderate injuries and who return to a previous job may find that they are "less organized" in their work. They are unable to shift their cognitive set and develop a planning strategy that would be appropriate for their work. These patients' spouses often complain that they are less attentive to them and have trouble separating out irrelevant bits of information when dealing with moderately complex tasks.

These types of disturbances reduce a person's efficiency and creativity and can greatly disturb interpersonal relationships, because it appears that the patient just does not care or is not motivated. Therapies for this type of cognitive disturbance have remained relatively sparse or nonexistent. These patients typically find jobs that require little initiative and are quite redundant, so that planning requirements are minimal and repetition skills are of major importance.

DISORDERS OF JUDGMENT AND PERCEPTION

While related to disorders of planning and abstract reasoning, additional disturbances in judgment and perception exist in traumatically brain-injured patients and should be separately identified. One of the most interesting disturbances centers around altered self-perceptions. Many brain-injured patients can recognize obvious physical disabilities, but they have trouble realistically appraising residual cognitive disturbances. They may admit they have "a little bit" of memory disturbance or a "minor" language problem but insist that they are able to return to work, when in fact their cognitive deficits clearly preclude this. When asked about self-perceived changes in personality or mood, they are prone to respond that no changes have taken place, despite relatives' protests to the contrary.

It appears, therefore, that realistic self-appraisal — one of the most highly integrated of all brain functions — is compromised after brain injury. Even subtle injuries of the brain may produce disturbances in this area. This phenomenon has been described or termed "denial of illness" by Weinstein and Kahn (1955). It is related to premorbid personality characteristics, but it also appears to have a clear neurological basis (see Chapter 3).

It has been our clinical impression that when altered self-awareness is mediated primarily by frontal lobe dysfunction, the patient can be substantially helped to improve self-perception. These patients are often inattentive, are concrete in their thinking, and misinterpret higher levels of information. In the context of intensive group interaction where information is given back in an objective and clear manner, these patients often improve. In contrast, with patients who show evidence of temporal lobe dysfunction with damage to associated deep-brain structures (e.g., amygdala), such therapies are usually less effective. The problem of altering self-awareness after brain injury, and its relationship to psychosocial adjustment, will be described in more detail below because of its major importance for rehabilitation outcome.

A second perceptual problem that head-injured patients can have centers on difficulties in perceiving the intentions or actions of others. These patients often show frank perceptual distortions on psychometric testing. Visual-spatial deficits and nonverbal memory disturbances are frequently present and compound the patient's inability to interpret affective information properly (see Prigatano and Pribram 1982). Ferguson et al. (1969) have demonstrated, for example, that temporal lobe seizure patients misread cartoons or humorous captions, misinterpreting them in a paranoid manner. Such paranoid ideations seem to reflect faulty perceptions as well as other cognitive deficits (see Leftoff 1983).

DISORDERS OF LEARNING AND MEMORY

Perhaps more than any other cognitive complaint, memory disturbances after traumatic brain injury are most well known. Russell (1971) described in scholarly detail the various forms of amnesia following closed-head injury. Schacter and Crovitz (1977) and Levin et al. (1982) reviewed much of the literature on memory disturbance after traumatic brain injury. Since the nature of the neuropathology in traumatic brain injury is so varied, it is

Table 1.1 Ischemic Brain Damage Associated with Severe Craniocerebral Trauma

	Cases with IBD[a] (138, 91% of total)
Hippocampus	122 (88%)
Basal ganglia	119 (86%)
Cerebral cortex (other than MOC)[b]	70 (51%)
Cerebellum	67 (49%)

Source: D. I. Graham, J. H. Adams, and D. Doyle, Ischemic brain damage in fatal nonmissile head injuries, *Journal of Neurological Sciences,* 1978, *39,* 213-234. Reprinted by permission of the journal.

[a] IBD = ischemic brain damage.
[b] MOC = medial occipital cortex.

not surprising that varying degrees and types of memory disturbances are observed after such injuries. The fact that hippocampal regions are at high risk for ischemic damage after significant brain injury helps explain why memory complaints are so common after traumatic head injury.

Patients who succumb following severe head injury show a high incidence of ischemic brain damage, particularly involving the hippocampus and basal ganglia. A study by Graham et al. (1978) showed that of the 91 percent of severe head-injury patients who had ischemic damage, 88 percent exhibited damage in the hippocampus and 86 percent exhibited damage in the basal ganglia. While memory is not "located" in the hippocampus, this structure appears to be important for the initial registration and later retrieval of information (see Butters 1979).

Memory skills have repeatedly been identified as important predictors of eventual work status. Bruckner and Randle (1972) compared working head-trauma patients to those not able to return to work. Some 65 percent (fifteen out of twenty-three) of the unemployed were considered to have memory impairment. In contrast, only 17 percent (four out of twenty-three) of the head-injured patients who were working were described as having memory difficulties.

Bond (1975) documented similar findings showing a clear relationship between memory disorder and work status. Weddell et al. (1980) reported that nonworking patients not only had significantly greater evidence of memory impairment but also showed a higher incidence of personality disturbance. In this regard, it is interesting to note that head-injured patients who were reported to have sustained personality changes (thirty-one out of forty-four) were also described as having greater memory disturbance. The intimate association of affective variables with cognitive variables is clearly demonstrated in this work. The same patients, it might be added, were likely to lose pretrauma friendships.

In the course of clinical rehabilitative work with these patients, one is impressed with the pervasiveness of memory disturbance. In the NRP, patients are asked daily throughout the entire program to state the name of each therapy hour and its purpose, but even with this repetition, several patients take four to eight weeks to learn successfully this simple information. Many standardized tests of memory fail to capture these and other real-life memory problems of traumatic head-injury patients. For example, forgetting where one parked the car, the name of a close friend, or the purpose of an important meeting is a frequent occurrence for such patients. These memory problems play havoc with day-to-day life adjustment.

While many attempts have been made to "remediate" memory disorders (Gianutsos and Gianutsos 1979; Gasparrini and Satz 1979; Prigatano 1983a), there are presently no therapies that make a "bad" memory "good." Helping the patient compensate for the memory disturbance (e.g., by having the patient use a pocket notebook) has been the most productive strategy for dealing with this difficulty. However, in many cases patients have personality disorders that add resistance to the use of compensatory techniques. A good deal of work must be focused on the psychotherapy of the personality disturbances in order to get these patients to use cognitive compensations.

DISORDERS OF THE SPEED OF INFORMATION-PROCESSING

Many craniocerebral trauma patients, especially those with brain-stem injuries, show decreased speed of information-processing. Such patients are slow in carrying out the simplest tasks (e.g., writing their name) and consequently keep others waiting. They require much more patience from family members and eventually are treated like children. This results in a great deal of discomfort in their interpersonal relationships. Gronwall and Sampson (1974) and Gronwall and Wrightson (1981) showed that even mild cerebral injuries can affect the speed at which information is processed. There is also a relationship between the length of posttraumatic amnesia (one measure of the severity of the injury) and later efficiency of information-processing.

In unpublished work with over one hundred traumatic head-injury patients seen at Presbyterian Hospital for diagnostic purposes, the speed of information-processing was related to the overall neuropsychological status and selected psychosocial difficulties. With the Trail Making Test, Part A, as a simple measure of the speed of psychomotor activity and information-processing, it was observed that this measure correlated highly with the Average Impairment Rating derived from the extended Halstead-Reitan Neuropsychological Test Battery (see Prigatano, Parsons, et al. 1983) ($r = +.65$, $p = .001$). Thus, the speed of simple information-processing that involved a motor response was highly related to overall problem-solving skills, perceptual ability, and higher-order tactual problem-solving abilities. Moreover, this simple measure of the speed of performance related in a positive way to the degree of social withdrawal as reported by relatives on patients by means of the Katz-R Adjustment Scale ($r = +.34$, $p = .002$). These data, and clinical experience, suggest that the basic capacity of the brain to process information rapidly has a profound impact on general adaptation and social adjustment. Patients who are slow in processing information often withdraw from the environment as a method of avoiding the catastrophic reaction. They choose a simple or predictable environment, as opposed to a complex and unpredictable one (see Chapter 3).

The question arises whether anything can be done to influence the recovery of this simple but important cognitive dimension. We observed with some surprise in our first outcome paper on the effectiveness of neuropsychological rehabilitation (Prigatano et al. 1984) that treated patients performed better on various timed tests than did controls. Since the NRP devotes one hour a day to increasing the speed of information-processing, during the cognitive retraining hour (see Chapter 6), it is possible that this rudimentary function can be subtly influenced with intensive retraining. In the light of how important this dimension appears to be for social functioning, further research is needed to explore this question carefully.

DISORDERS OF COMMUNICATION (APHASIC AND NONAPHASIC)

Like memory disturbances, varying types of communication disorders exist after serious traumatic brain injury. When injury occurs to the left, or dominant, cerebral hemisphere, frank aphasic symptomatology emerges. Often, however, no clear aphasic syndrome exists; there may be instead a mixture of aphasic disturbances. Several months postinjury, when the classic aphasic signs either disappear or are greatly diminished, there are still residual signs of anomia and reduced word fluency (Levin et al. 1976, 1981). Dresser et al. (1973) reported that in brain-injured patients who show residual aphasic disturbances there is a significant impact on employability. On follow-up, only 60 percent of aphasic patients were employed, and as the severity of the aphasia increased, the incidence of employment decreased.

In addition to the aphasic disturbances, nonaphasic language disturbances are present, and exceedingly important for social adaptation. Described in more detail in the next chapter, these problems include talkativeness or verbal expansiveness, tangentiality of thought in conversational speech, and the use of peculiar words or phrases. Some brain-injured patients simply talk too much. They do not know when to stop and give others a turn to speak. This can be extremely irritating to other people and often results in sarcastic remarks from those having to deal with such overtalkative individuals. Oddy et al. (1978b) showed a persistent positive correlation between talkativeness or verbal expansiveness of patients (as judged by the Katz-R Adjustment Scale) with the patients' relatives' mood disturbance six to twelve months postinjury.

Unpublished data with traumatically brain-injured patients seen at Presbyterian Hospital shows a correlation between verbal expansiveness and neuropsychological and psychosocial difficulties. The verbal expansiveness measure (from the Katz-R Adjustment Scale) was significantly correlated with errors on the Halstead Category Test ($r = +.28$, $p = .04$, $N = 49$). Overtalkativeness may be related to frontal lobe dysfunction, since this test is purportedly sensitive to such disturbances (Halstead 1947). More striking, however, was the relationship of verbal expansiveness to the general measure of psychopathology on the Katz Adjustment Scale ($r = +.66$, $p = .001$, $N = 116$). It has been our clinical impression that the more anxious and uninhibited patients are generally more talkative.

A common problem in traumatically head-injured patients is that of tangentiality (see Levin et al. 1979). This disturbance is difficult to objectify and measure. Often the surface structure of the language output is normal but conceptual confusion is obvious, as reflected in problems of word selection, loose connection of thoughts and ideas, impaired abstract reasoning, and a strong tendency to stray from the core message. This problem can be seen in the written and spoken speech of traumatically head-injured patients. It often gives the listener the impression that "something" is wrong with this person, but one cannot easily identify what is wrong. A detailed example of this problem will be presented in the next chapter, on nonaphasic language disturbances. We say here only that it has been our clinical experience that this type of disturbance can be modified, within limits. Given intensive group therapy in which patients are asked to engage in a variety of cognitive tasks, there can be an enhanced awareness of faulty conceptualization and verbal output. Slowly, many patients can modify their language, given this immediate and repetitive feedback (see Chapter 5).

A final nonaphasic language disturbance is the use of peculiar phraseology. Patients may refer to themselves in the third person or use words in a grammatically peculiar fashion. For example, one patient used to refer to herself as "Sharon K" when in direct communication with another individual. Weinstein and Kahn (1955) suggest that this type of disturbance in linguistic function may be associated with amnestic disorder and/or problems in self-awareness.

Unrealistic Self-appraisal after Brain Injury

Unrealistic self-appraisal following traumatic brain injury may play a major role in problems of psychosocial adjustment for many individuals

(Ben-Yishay et al. 1981; Prigatano and Fordyce, in press). Conflict with family members, poor vocational decisions, and poor motivation for rehabilitation frequently relate directly to a diminished self-awareness of deficits that can exist for months or years posttrauma. As with other serious disabilities, denial of the effects of brain injury can be viewed as an ego-protective coping strategy. It is also clear, however, that diminished awareness of disability following brain injury can reflect neurologically based information-processing deficits. This is most floridly represented in the anosognosia for left hemiplegia following right hemisphere infarct. It is also seen in the confusional state that accompanies posttraumatic amnesia and the more advanced stages of some dementing disorders. In the case of anosognosia for left hemiplegia, a spectrum of related disorders have been identified, including hemi-inattention, hemi-akinesia, allesthesia, hemispatial neglect, and anosodiaphoria (Heilman 1979). It has recently been theorized that the central information-processing deficit underlying these disorders is a state of generalized cortical hypoarousal and an accompanying diminished alerting or orienting response to novel stimulation (Bear 1983; Heilman 1979). The right inferior parietal lobule, dorsal limbic structures, certain thalamic nuclei, the dorsolateral frontal cortex, and brain-stem reticular activating system pathways seem to form an arousal-orienting system. Lesions in any of these structures appear to lead to anosognosia-like disorders (Heilman 1979). These neuroanatomical areas, particularly the frontal poles and the brain stem (Ommaya and Gennerelli 1974), are at risk for injury in severe traumatic head injury.

Prior to addressing the particular rehabilitation needs of a chronic traumatically head-injured individual, it is important to assess the extent to which the patient is aware of the specific cognitive deficits. Motivated participation in cognitive retraining activities presupposes awareness of the particular target problem (Diller and Gordon 1981). It is also important to understand whether the negation of disability reflects primarily neurologically based information-processing deficits or the more psychologically based "denial of illness." Typically, both components are present (Weinstein and Kahn 1955).

We have attempted to measure diminished self-awareness following traumatic brain injury within a larger framework of assessing the different perspectives on disability that patients, relatives, and rehabilitation staff bring to the rehabilitation setting (Roueche and Fordyce 1983). This is accomplished by having patients, relatives, and staff members rate the patient's ability to perform a variety of everyday behaviors on a thirty-item five-point behavioral rating scale (see Appendix A and Appendix B). The majority of patients seen in rehabilitation tend to rate themselves as generally more competent, compared with the ratings of family members and rehabilitation staff members. The magnitude of these differences provides some quantification of the tendency to minimize disability. The social-psychological aspects of this method are clear and are highlighted by the fact that family members tend to see the patient as more competent than the rehabilitation staff does. Comparisons of the ratings of behavioral competency with standardized neuropsychological test scores and emotional functioning as assessed by the Minnesota Multiphasic Personality Inventory (MMPI) have been undertaken for twenty-three patients seen in rehabilitation. Differences in perceived competency between patients and staff members are positively correlated with the level of neuropsychological impairment and negatively correlated with the magnitude of emotional distress as assessed by the MMPI. These preliminary findings suggest that the greater the tendency for the patient to minimize disability relative to staff members, the greater the patient's level of neuropsychological impairment and the less the self-reported emotional distress. These data corroborate clinical impressions that in a group of head-injured patients some portion of the variance in the tendency to minimize disability may reflect impaired self-awareness that parallels other residual cognitive deficits. In addition, however, minimization of disability may also help shelter individuals from excessive psychological turmoil. Those who rate themselves as most competent relative to staff members' ratings tend not to endorse heightened emotional distress on the MMPI.

Further refinement is needed to understand the extent to which impaired self-awareness is present in patients presenting for rehabilitation a number of years posttrauma. The nature of intervention methods depends greatly on how much the patient appears to know about his or her disability and, equally important, whether the patient's level of understanding reflects an apparent lack of self-awareness or psychological denial. In the former, awareness training may be an appropriate rehabilitation target, although subsequent denial may be a by-product of such activity. In the latter, awareness training may lead to resistance and heightened emotional distress.

The Problem of Unemployment

We have already noted that cognition or cognitive dysfunction cannot be adequately defined or studied devoid of the concepts of emotion and motivation. Nowhere is this more obvious than in the study of the long-term problems of adjustment of brain-injured patients, particularly relating to employment. Research in England by Michael Oddy and associates (Weddell et al. 1980; Oddy et al. 1978*a*, 1978*b*) emphasizes that patients with severe head injury have difficulty maintaining gainful employment, keeping pretrauma relationships, and generally existing adequately within the context of previous family life. In the NRP, it has been clear that notable changes of body image occur, as well as expected reduction in self-esteem and enhanced dependency on family members and welfare systems. Some family members seem to foster this dependency without being fully aware of it.

In this section, studies that deal with identifying the variables that predict employment either after brain injury or associated with brain injury will be reviewed. These studies, for the most part, employ both neuropsychological and personality measures. They repeatedly demonstrate that it is a *combination* of cognitive and affective variables which influences the important outcome of whether patients return to gainful employment.

Dennerll et al. (1966) investigated a wide variety of neurological and psychological predictors of employability in patients with epilepsy. Unemployed patients had "mild impairment of rapid alternate motions and definite problems in imitating motions." They showed greater cognitive impairment and difficulties getting along with others than did the employed patients. The inability to cope effectively with interpersonal demands was specifically identified as an important factor for unsuccessful employment.

Heaton et al. (1978) studied neuropsychological and personality test results in a large group of varied brain-injured patients and related their scores to employment status. The Average Impairment Rating, a summary statistic of overall neuropsychological functioning, reliably separated employed brain-injured patients from unemployed patients. It did not, however, discriminate between part-time employed and full-time employed individuals. The speed of information-processing skills and the ability to learn new information (as measured by the Wechsler Adult Intelligence Scale [WAIS] Digit Symbol subtest) had similar discriminatory power. Pure speed of motor movement (e.g., speed of finger tapping) reliably separated all patient groups: the faster the performance, the greater the likelihood of employability. Even part-time and full-time employed patients were separated on this simple speed measure. This reaffirms the importance of speed, motor function, and the general ability to process information for ultimate psychosocial outcome. In the same study, the self-reported degree of depression separated all groups equally. This is interesting, since many behavioral methods have been established to treat depressive disorder.

In a second report, Newnan et al. (1978) related the same test scores to whether patients were chronically unemployed and their actual wage level. The Average Impairment Rating correlated significantly with both measures, although the magnitude of the relationship was modest ($r = +.47$ and $+.37$ respectively). It is interesting to note that concerns over bodily function (the hypochondriasis scale on the MMPI) and measures of anxiety (the hysteria scale) had only modest relationships with chronic unemployment ($r = +.22$ and $r = +.29$ respectively).

Dikmen and Morgan (1980) added the important observation that premorbid occupational status also predicted employment. In a group of epileptic patients, two-thirds of the unemployed patients studied had a history of being unskilled laborers. Two studies by Rimel et al. (1981, 1982) reaffirmed the same findings. In mild head injury, a greater portion of patients unemployed three months postinjury were unskilled laborers, compared with the working patients, who were executives or had skilled positions pretrauma. Some 42 percent of moderately impaired head-injured patients (Glasgow Coma Scale score of 9–13) were unskilled laborers or chronically unemployed. These observations emphasize the importance of premorbid factors in predicting psychosocial outcome for this patient group.

Finally, two studies pointed out the importance of personality variables for eventual employment. Weddell et al. (1980) reported that head-injured patients with greater personality change (often enhanced irritability) were less likely to return to work and had fewer interests and fewer friends. In addition, they were clearly more dependent on their families. Prigatano et al. (1984) reported that head-injured patients who returned to work after intensive neuropsychological rehabilitation showed greater improvement on overall measures of psychopathology, hyperactivity, and social stability. These patients also showed signs of greater improvement in simple speed of information-processing and new learning.

Summary

This chapter has described, primarily from a rehabilitation point of view, the major cognitive disturbances seen in traumatically head-injured patients several months postinjury. These disturbances have been classified into six broad categories: problems of attention and concentration, initiation and planning, judgment and perception, learning and memory, speed of information-processing, and communication. While these difficulties overlap, problems seem to cluster according to these dimensions. The problems of unrealistic self-appraisal after brain injury are especially common and important after traumatic brain injury.

Rehabilitation programs, whether they foster intensive neuropsychological rehabilitation activities or more traditional methods of treatment, must deal with these problems if the patients are eventually to return to gainful employment. Bond and Brooks (1976) emphasized that it is typically the cognitive and personality disturbances of traumatically head-injured patients that are neglected in the rehabilitation of these individuals, and yet these are by far the most important predictors of eventual (work) outcome.

While many clinicians have been pessimistic, saying that treating these cognitive and related personality disturbances is futile, it has been our experience that intensive rehabilitative efforts can substantially help many individuals. Frequently the problem is helping the patient and the family identify the cognitive strengths and weaknesses after injury and teaching them methods of compensating for those deficits. The utilization of compensatory techniques is not an easy process, and existing personality disturbances in patient and family members may preclude the use of these techniques. Consequently, dealing with these patients from a psychotherapeutic point of view is an important complement to working with them in the identification and remediation of cognitive disturbances.

CHAPTER 2
Nonaphasic Language Disturbances after Brain Injury

George P. Prigatano, James R. Roueche, and David J. Fordyce

Disturbances of brain physiology can interfere with language function. The most commonly studied language disorders after brain injury are the aphasic syndromes, which frequently occur following discrete vascular disturbances of the left cerebral hemisphere (Benson 1979). Severe craniocerebral trauma, which often produces nondiscrete, bilateral cerebral disturbance, can also interfere with language function. Both generalized and specific linguistic disorders have been noted following such trauma (Levin et al. 1981).

In many cases, after cognitive and aphasic disturbances have partially recovered, subtle difficulties in linguistic function persist. The so-called nonaphasic language disturbances greatly hamper a patient's social adjustment and can interfere with rehabilitation efforts, but no specific therapeutic strategies for dealing with them have yet emerged. This chapter describes three nonaphasic language disturbances associated with significant craniocerebral trauma. An initial therapeutic strategy for dealing with them will be described in Chapters 5 and 6.

When injury to the adult left cerebral hemisphere takes place through trauma or any other means, disturbance in language function is typical. The term *aphasia* is usually applied to language disturbances where a generalized language impairment that crosses all language modalities (i.e., speaking, reading, and writing) is present. This disturbance presumably reflects a primary difficulty in the symbolic mode of information-processing and thereby interferes with communication. The term *aphasia* is usually not applied when there is a generalized dementing condition or severe amnestic disturbance that secondarily impinges on language function.

An earlier version of this chapter will appear in a *Language Sciences* monograph (in press).

While Luria (1966) showed that language disturbances can occur from lesions throughout the left hemisphere, two classic aphasic syndromes are recognized. The first is Broca's aphasia, which results from lesions of the left frontal gyrus, typically producing a nonfluent language output while sparing auditory comprehension. The second is Wernicke's aphasia, which results from lesions in the superior left temporal gyrus, producing a fluent language output with perseverative paraphasia and limitations in comprehension. Benson (1979) described these well-known forms of aphasia, in addition to other types of aphasic disturbance that have been recognized but are not necessarily universally accepted: conduction aphasia, transcortical motor aphasia, transcortical sensory aphasia, global aphasia, and anomic or amnestic aphasia.

The phrase "nonaphasic disorders of language" refers to disturbances in communication in which there is no classic aphasic syndrome present. In these situations, nondominant as well as dominant cerebral hemisphere lesions may be present. Geschwind (1964) noted, for example, that neurological patients with diffuse brain disease have problems in the appropriate use of syntax in addition to anomic difficulties. While these patients are not classically "aphasic" as outlined by the recognized syndromes of aphasia, their language output does reflect inadequacies in communication.

Levin and colleagues (1979, 1981) noted the great variability of aphasic and nonaphasic language disturbances in closed-head-injury patients. While conversational speech and ability to comprehend recover in many such patients, there are frequently residual paraphasic errors, word-finding (i.e., fluency) difficulties, and varying degrees of anomia. Such patients often show "tangential, fragmented speech not attributed to aphasia and deficient cognitive filtering of irrelevant material" (Levin et al. 1981: 417).

Other authors have also been impressed with these language disorders following trauma. Weinstein and Keller (1963) reported on naming errors in patients with right, left, and bilateral deeply seated lesions. Some of these patients had traumatic brain injuries. The left hemisphere patients showed phonemic and symbolic coding errors. The right hemisphere patients and patients with diffuse and deep brain lesions made few naming errors, but their errors seemed to reflect problems of personal orientation to the environment. They reflected disturbances in perceived social context, while formal linguistic components of language production appeared to be preserved.

Lackner (1982) noted that, some twenty years posttrauma, head-injured patients may still have difficulties resolving linguistic ambiguities despite the resolution of an earlier aphasia. Finally, Luria (1977) noted that lesions of the thalamus can produce so-called quasi-aphasic disturbances; that is, a disorder in filtering out irrelevant material or ideas in a given communication is seen. This seems to be secondary to disturbances in vigilance and ability to sustain attention and activation. Marin et al. (1979) suggested that such brain lesions affect speech and memory in a manner similar to fatigue and toxic drug states. In both instances there seems to be a certain degree of "cortical inefficiency" that indirectly influences language production.

The Problem of Talkativeness

Some traumatically head-injured patients are restless, disinhibited, and talkative several months after the acute period following trauma. Forty-eight consecutive closed-head-injury patients, referred for clinical neuropsychological assessment, were studied regarding the presence or absence of restlessness and talkativeness. The patients ranged in age from 15 to 57 years, with a mean age of 27.5 years (standard deviation $[SD] = 9.5$). They were predominantly males (43 men, 5 females) with a high school education (mean education was 12.2 years; $SD = 3.1$). The patients were studied an average of 16 months postinjury, but the time since injury varied from 1 to 81 months.

As part of their clinical assessment, the patients' relatives completed the Katz-R Adjustment Scale (see McSweeny et al. 1982 for a description of this scale). The scale lists several behavioral characteristics on which the relatives rate the patient, including "is restless" and "talks too much." The patient can be rated by the relatives as having this problem "almost never," "only sometimes," "often," or "almost always." Patients whose relatives indicated that they "almost never" or "only sometimes" showed the behavioral problem were grouped first. The patients who were rated by their relatives as "often" or "almost always" demonstrating the problem were classified in a second group. Twenty-two of the patients were rated by their relatives as "not restless," while 26 were rated as "restless." Of these 48 patients studied, only 8 (or 16 percent) were judged by their relatives as being too talkative. All of these 8 patients, however, were judged as being "restless."

Compared with the remaining forty nontalkative patients, the talkative closed-head-injury patients generally did not differ in age, education, length of coma, chronicity of illness, or neuropsychological status. For example, there was no difference in their WAIS or WAIS-R Vocabulary, Block Design, or Digit Symbol subtest scores. While their average impairment ratings, derived from the extended Halstead-Reitan Neuropsychological Test Battery, showed no difference between the two groups (see Prigatano, Parsons et al. 1983, for a description of this measure), a modest correlation between talkativeness and errors on the Halstead Category Test were observed (see Chapter 1).

The talkative group was judged to have clearly more emotional

Table 2.1 Katz-Relatives' Form Ratings of 48 Brain-injured Patients Classified as "Talkative" or "Not Talkative" (Mean Z Scores)

Subtest	Not Talkative ($N = 40$)	Talkative ($N = 8$)
Belligerence	1.41	2.86[a]
Verbal expansiveness	1.31	2.28[a]
Negativism	1.79	2.62[a]
Helplessness	2.32[a]	2.09[a]
Suspiciousness	2.34[a]	3.64[a]
Anxiety	0.98	3.05[a]
Withdrawal/depression	2.89[a]	2.62[a]
General psychopathology	5.04[a]	4.81[a]
Nervousness	2.37[a]	2.08[a]
Confusion	1.12	1.76
Bizzareness	0.75	1.89
Hyperactivity	2.04[a]	2.34[a]
Stability	−1.04	−4.38[a]

[a] Z value at p .05 level or greater.

distress. Table 2.1 shows the Katz-R adjustment ratings of "talkative" and "nontalkative" patients. The talkative patients had numerous behavioral difficulties, including heightened belligerence, negativism, helplessness, suspiciousness, anxiety, withdrawal and depression, and other forms of psychopathology. These data are interesting because they suggest that this nonaphasic communication disturbance may have more to do with the feeling or emotional characteristics of the patient than with their cognitive deficits per se. The finding is in keeping with findings of Weinstein and Keller (1963) and Weinstein and Kahn (1955), who noted the importance of affective disturbance in producing nonaphasic linguistic difficulties in traumatic head-injury patients.

The Problem of Tangentiality

As was noted by Levin et al. (1979), significant craniocerebral trauma often results in tangential expression of ideas. This disturbance, which can occur in both spoken and written forms, is relatively common but difficult to objectify and study. While the surface structure of language output appears to be intact, conceptual confusion is obvious and is reflected in problems of poor word selection, loose connection of thoughts and ideas, impairment in abstract thinking, and a strong tendency to stray from the core message or topic.

The following is an example of a written narrative made by one of our patients who shows this problem of tangentiality. The patient is a thirty-four-year-old hospital executive who suffered a severe traumatic head injury approximately two years ago. He was asked to write a paragraph in response to the question "What would you like to do at the end of your rehabilitation program?" The patient wrote the following:

> My first choice is to go back to work at the hospital. This would be hard for me to do, because they have hired someone to take my place. I liked the work. I was there for over 5 years. I also would like to go to a sheltered workshop. This would be good, but it has to have transportation to the place and to home. The transportation would have to be a bus, because I do not have a driver's license. I was to have it renewed last year, but that was not done. To get a driver's license, I will need to take the written and the driver's exam. The workshop will help me control my temper, which is bad for me. I get mad easily and this is because of my brain injury. All that I can recall is that I was knocked out for 3 weeks. I did the recovery at Mercy ICU. I had the car accident on my way to the hospital for a personnel directors meeting. The workshop might have been in Austin, Texas. This means I will be away from home, which I would miss very much. I miss not being at home. I would like to work in the yard and work on the cars, especially washing and waxing them. This I have not done for over 2 years.

This description highlights a number of common characteristics in the tangential thinking of brain-injured patients. The patient begins with a description of what he wants, namely, to return to his previous employment. He also considers a second option, that of going to a sheltered workshop. He then begins to become tangential. He starts to talk about his transportation needs. From there he begins to talk about his desire to have a driver's license and what he would have to do to get a license. His thoughts then go back to the sheltered workshop setting. He is aware that he has problems with temper and that this problem is the result of brain injury. From there he begins to talk about how his brain injury occurred, what was happening to him at the time, and so on. He then returns to the topic of the sheltered workshop and where it might be. Finally, the patient ends with a description of his loneliness and his desire to stay in the Oklahoma City area.

This type of tangential thinking and verbalization reflects a fragmented thought process, the intrusion of ideas, and the confusion of the melting together of concepts and feelings in the patient's mind. This was present even though the patient was able to spell all the words accurately, use fairly good grammar and sentence structure, and had in front of him his written narrative, that is, he could read over what he had written and correct it if he wished. The problem therefore appears to be at the conceptual level of language despite relatively intact written linguistic skills.

The neuropsychological examination of this patient revealed that he is oriented to time and place but has notable problems in short-term memory. His intelligence, as measured by psychometric tests, reflected low-average scores (Verbal IQ = 89, Performance IQ = 87, Full Scale IQ = 87). Verbal reasoning was mildly impaired (Similarities Scale score = 8). The patient becomes quite easily confused when he is asked to shift his cognitive set. For example, on the Trail Making Test, Part B, his completion time was 178 seconds and he made two errors. Assessment of language function reveals difficulty in naming (he scored in the severely defective range of the Visual Naming subtest of the Multilingual Aphasia Examination). He also had problems in sentence repetition (defective range) and rapid word retrieval or association (defective range). None of these deficits, however, was obvious in casual conversation with the patient. Other measures of language function were generally within normal limits. The problems in repetition demonstrated by this patient seem to be related to short-term memory difficulties, as opposed to the paraphasic disturbance in repeating auditory inputs seen in some aphasic disturbances. This case highlights the association of core neuropsychological impairments with the tangential thinking and communication seen in closed-head-injury patients. In addition, one must further question the relationship and impact of specific linguistic impairments on this phenomenon.

Future linguistic assessment of tangential verbalizations after closed-head injury might follow the example provided by Rochester et al. (1977). These researchers showed that schizophrenic verbalizations were very difficult for listeners to follow because the patients typically made statements that required the listener to search for information that was never clearly given by the speaker. The patients also provided relatively few conjunctive links between clauses, which made the listening task a difficult one.

The Phenomenon of Peculiar Phraseology

A third nonaphasic language disturbance is that of using unusual or peculiar phraseology. Weinstein et al. (1962) recognized that closed-head-injury patients with amnestic disturbances are prone to talk about themselves in the "third person" and use "various forms of metaphoric expression" (p. 265). He felt that this reflected an underlying disturbance in the sense of contact with or awareness of the environment. While not an extremely common problem several months postinjury, this phenomenon does exist and should be addressed in neuropsychologically oriented rehabilitation.

One example of this phenomenon is seen in the verbalizations of a thirty-seven-year-old woman who received a significant cerebral and brain-stem contusion with clear left hemisphere signs (e.g., presence of residual right hemiparesis) but with the absence of dysphasia. Despite essentially normal CT scan findings (see Fig. 2.1) and minor bilateral slowing on the electroencephalogram (Fig. 2.2), she had major neuropsychological disturbance several months postinjury.

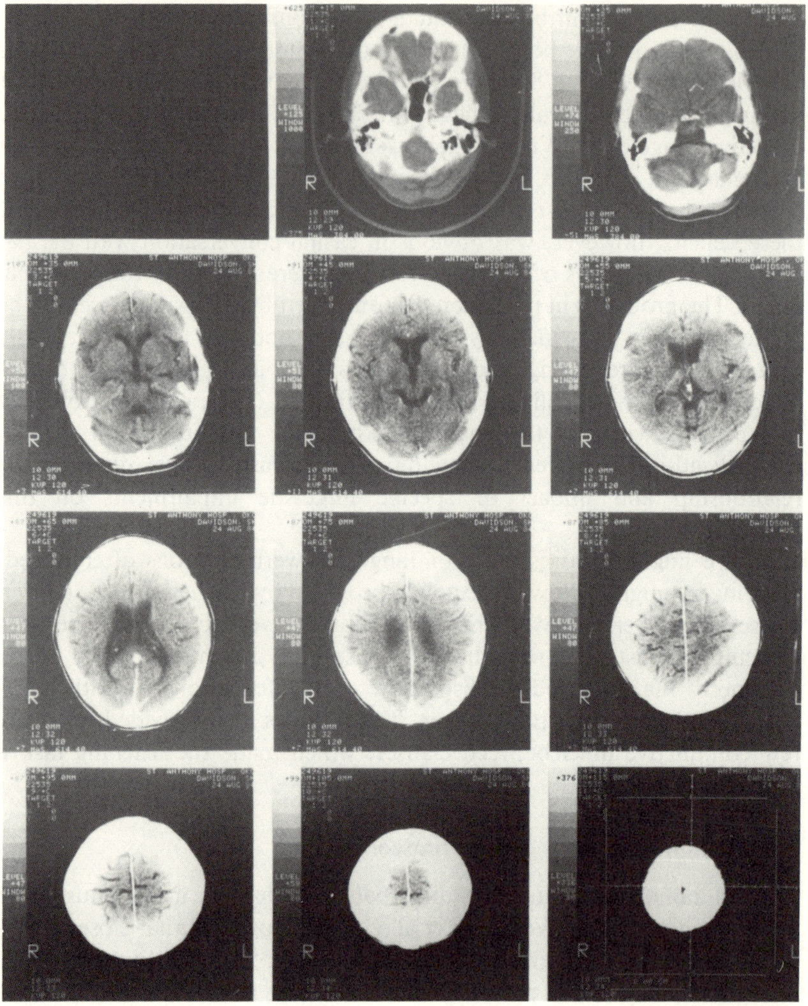

Figure 2.1. Reportedly Normal CT Scan in a Young Adult Female Patient with Significant Neuropsychological Sequelae after Severe Craniocerebral Trauma. Courtesy of the Radiology Department, St. Anthony Hospital, Oklahoma City, Okla.

This once productive and socially energetic individual became severely amnestic and progressively isolated from family members and friends. She would confabulate, and this was very upsetting to those who lived with her and knew her in the past. She became more and more paranoid and denied the severity of her memory problems. Her attempts to explain her social isolation were usually based on the belief that because she was in the

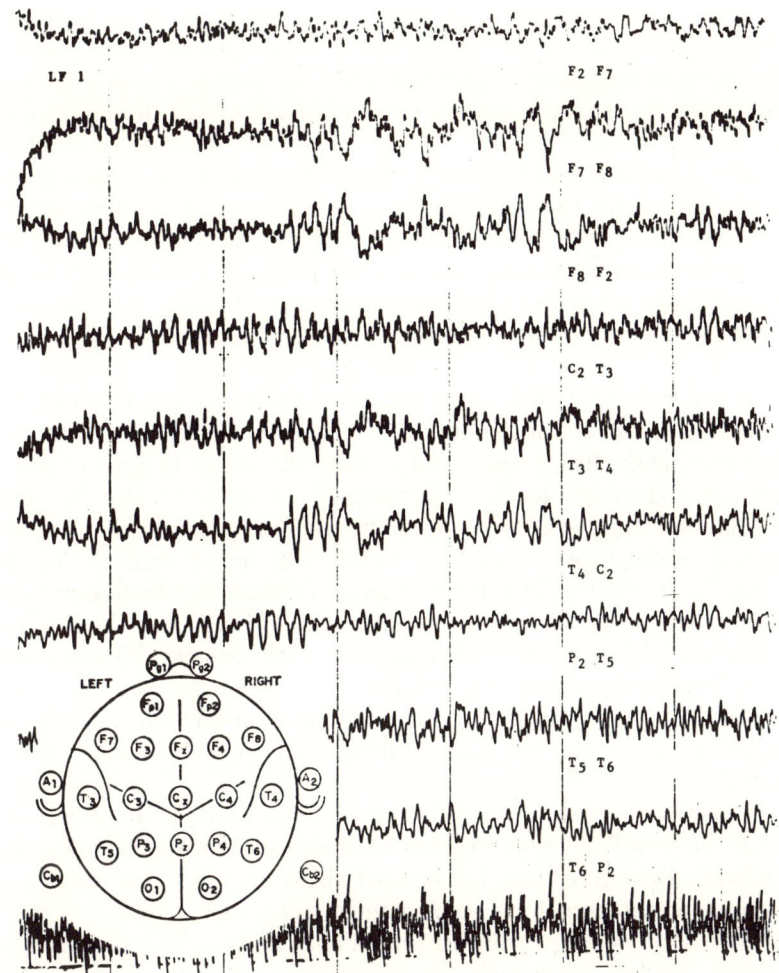

Figure 2.2. EEG Recording in the Same Patient Several Months Postinjury. Courtesy of Richard Carpenter, M.D., Oklahoma City, Okla.

hospital for so long and not involved in family and social matters, people had simply gone about their business and developed a life exclusive of her.

She could not face the fact that her memory difficulties, confabulation, periodic angry outbursts, and paranoid ideation were the real cause of her social difficulties. When asked, for example, why she felt that her husband did not treat her better (in reality he treated her very well), she answered: "I was out so long he handles things the other way." This last phrase, "handles things the other way," was her attempt at saying that he no longer treats her in the same manner as he did before the injury. When asked further why others do not actively involve her in social interactions, she made the following statement: "Like sometimes I am far else, being in the way. Even — I don't need to comment. I always hear them say 'he and the girls, and he and the girls and her.'" The patient was attempting to make the point that she does not even need to comment on the fact that she is treated as if she does not exist when she is in the presence of her husband and daughters. The phrase "he and the girls" refers to her belief that others talk only to her husband and the daughters and purposely exclude her from the conversation. When they recognize her presence, they use "her" in a pejorative manner, as opposed to calling her by her first name as they used to do.

Formal language testing of this patient on the Multilingual Aphasia Examination reveals essentially normal language functioning, although there are some subtle difficulties. She does have difficulties in naming and in repeating sentences, as did the previous patient. She also has mild difficulties in rapid word retrieval, yet her auditory comprehension, speech fluency, reading, spelling, and articulation skills are all within the normal limits. The difficulties in sentence repetition appeared to be related to her short-term memory disturbance (see Lackner 1974). Her intelligence was within the average range (Verbal IQ = 101, Performance IQ = 92), with clear impairment in memory functioning (Wechsler Memory Quotient = 79). This woman's speed and flexibility in thinking was also reduced, as noted on the Trail Making Test (A = 47 seconds, B = 95 seconds).

The patient frequently referred to herself in the third person. When talking about herself, she would use her first name and middle initial. This has gradually disappeared, but her peculiar choice of words and phrases remains as it has been for several months and makes it difficult for the listener to follow the meaning of her communications. This woman occasionally becomes tangential, but this occurs less frequently than the peculiar phrases. The listener's primary problem is understanding the meaning of the phrases and words she uses in combination. While the basic message can be gleaned from the patient's redundant narrative, the listener is forced to repeat to her the essence of her communication to reaffirm the meaning of her comments. This kind of behavioral problem seems to reflect both cognitive and emotional difficulties involving the patient's view of herself in relationship to the environment.

An additional example of nonaphasic language disturbance demonstrates peculiar phraseology and word order. This patient, a twenty-one-year-old male who suffered severe bilateral frontal injury with associated basal ganglia disturbance, was asked to respond to the question "How would you resolve a situation in which the loud music of a neighborhood teenager was keeping a family's children awake at night?" His response was: "Either call their neighbors or knock on the door to the parents of the child, answer and tell them there is every night or most nights, there is a loud music coming from their children's or child's, their teenage child's car in the driveway and they can't, their children, the Edwards' children, can't sleep in their room which is near the music because of the loud noise." This sequence appears to reflect a basic conceptual understanding of both the problem and the proposed solution. The prominent feature in this narrative, however, is the patient's repeated refinement or revision of statements with frequent repetition of detail. To the listener these refinements are not necessary, but for the patient the repetition seems to help clarify the point. Despite the fragmented construction, this patient did not become tangential in his thinking, as seen in the sample of our first patient. The problems in phraseology do not seem to reflect any personality or affective disturbance as seen in the last sample, but rather seem to reflect cognitive processing difficulties.

This patient's neuropsychological profile is characterized by average memory functioning (Wechsler Memory Quotient = 100), decreased speed and flexibility in information processing (Trails A = 112 seconds, B = 303 seconds), and low general intelligence (Verbal IQ = 90, Performance IQ = 63). This man's communication skill is quite functional, but specific linguistic limitations are noted in naming, rapid word retrieval, and sentence repetition.

These three cases are characteristic of the nonaphasic disturbances. Each demonstrates clear neuropsychological impairment but functional communication in the presence of specific residual linguistic impairment. In addition, the qualitative influence of the patient's sense of contact with or awareness of the environment (Weinstein et al. 1962) seems to play a role in communication, as noted in our second case.

These preliminary observations of the communication difficulties seen following traumatic head injury suggest the need for more complete understanding of the interaction of affective state, linguistic skill, and cognitive functioning in this population.

Summary

This chapter has focused on three nonaphasic language disturbances observed following significant craniocerebral trauma: the problems of talkativeness, tangential verbalizations, and the use of peculiar phraseology. These disturbances greatly compromise a patient's ability to communicate effectively in both social and vocational settings and may result in significant social isolation or unemployment. While a more complete understanding of these problems is needed, there appears to be a clear association with difficulties in linguistic performance, disturbances in shifting cognitive set, and problems with memory and emotional/motivational adjustment.

CHAPTER 3
Personality and Psychosocial Consequences of Brain Injury

George P. Prigatano

Brain lesions of various types produce alterations in personality, but they are frequently overlooked because they lack neurological diagnostic utility (e.g., lesion localization) and are difficult to measure objectively. Moreover, a patient's preexisting personality characteristics interact with neuropathologically mediated changes in cognition and affect to yield variable patterns of personality disturbances. Thus, descriptions such as "frontal lobe personality syndrome" are doomed to be oversimplified (Blumer and Benson 1975) and confusing to both clinicians and researchers. As the connecting neural circuitry between limbic structures and the cerebral hemispheres is identified, greater understanding of personality changes after brain injury will occur and a true "neurology of emotion" will be possible (see Bear 1983).

The importance of personality disturbances following brain injury is obvious to rehabilitation therapists and family members of the patient. Having to deal with these patients on a day-to-day basis is difficult, and their personality characteristics either lessen the work load or substantially increase it. Patients who seem depressed and unmotivated often frustrate therapists and receive minimal therapy or inappropriate therapy. Those who are paranoid and have trouble controlling their temper may simply be eliminated from rehabilitative programs on the basis that they are "management problems." Yet these affective disturbances are frequently as neurologically based as aphasia and hemiplegia. In addition, there are also affective problems that are part of the reaction the patient experiences when attempting to cope with disabilities, as Goldstein (1942) pointed out years ago. These later disturbances are potentially amenable to change if

---

An earlier version of this chapter will appear in M. Meier, L. Diller, and A. Benton, eds., *Neuropsychological Rehabilitation* (London: Churchill Livingstone, in press). Reprinted by permission of the publisher.

the rehabilitation therapist can teach the patient more efficient means of coping. This has been one major goal of our intensive neuropsychological rehabilitation program for young adult brain-injured patients (see Chapter 6).

While various models of personality that generate interesting concepts concerning the nature of psychopathology have appeared (see Freedman et al. 1976), these models often do not relate directly to what is known about brain function. When attempts have been made to do this (Pribram and Gill 1976), the result is often more theoretical in nature than clinically useful.

Neuropsychological Considerations of Personality

Personality is defined as patterns of emotional and motivational responses that develop over the life of the organism; are highly influenced by early life experiences; are modifiable, but not easily changed, by behavioral or teaching methods; and greatly influence (and are influenced by) cognitive processes. In humans, these patterns of emotional and motivational responses are in part self-recognized, but they may remain outside the individual's realm of conscious awareness. Others, who are familiar with the individual's daily behavioral characteristics, may recognize emotional and motivational responses that the person may not be fully aware of or able to report subjectively. Finally, the form of a given emotional and/or motivational response is highly dependent on the environmental consequences as well as on the biological state of the organism. This definition draws heavily from the work of Pribram (1971), Freud (1924), Jung (1964), various "social biologists" (e.g., Timbergen 1953 and Lorenz 1966), Simon (1967), Goldstein (1942), and Harry Stack Sullivan (1953). As such, biological, psychological, and psychosocial constructs are inevitably involved in defining personality.

Neuropsychology can aid in defining what emotions and motivations are and the neural structures involved in sustaining them. Also, the disturbing effects of various brain lesions on the balance between affect and cognition can be understood by studying neuropsychologic mechanisms (e.g., Prigatano and Pribram 1981). Eventually a neuropsychological model of the underlying structures and dynamics involved in personality should become a reality.

Feelings are the most rudimentary, generalized, and differentiated perceptions of internal bodily states. By nature they have an intensity or an arousal dimension to them (Lindsley 1970). Core brain receptors involved in the central nervous system's regulation of the organism's metabolic and endocrine functions are probably responsible for the initial or "crude" sensation of feeling states. These core brain receptors for temperature, thirst, hunger, pain, and respiration are localized in the brain stem and are near the midline ventricular system involving hypothalamic and midline thalamic nuclei (see Pribram 1971).

If feelings can be considered the basic representation for homeostatic states of the organism, the terms *emotion* and *motivation* can be used to refer to more complex and refined feeling states that incorporate basic homeostasis but also go beyond it. *Motivation* refers to the complex feeling states that parallel hierarchical goal-seeking behavior (Simon 1967). As such, it can be described as the arousal component of behavior which sees to it that a plan of action is developed and executed. In Simon's (1967) information-processing terms, motivation controls attention and thereby influences learning by influencing which program will be followed. A program here is defined simply as a series of steps that are taken in order to achieve a goal (Miller et al. 1960).

Using Simon's (1967) model, *emotion,* on the other hand, refers to the complex feeling states that parallel an interruption of whatever ongoing goal-seeking behaviors or programs are engaged. According to Simon, emotion interrupts an ongoing process, particularly when stimuli enter the perceptual world, which must be attended to for survival value. In humans, attention to the activities of other humans is especially important for survival, and thus emotion is crucial and indispensable in human social interaction. While there are certainly other models of motivation and emotion, this system has appeal for the neuropsychologically oriented clinician.

Schacter and Singer (1962) eloquently showed that the cognitive appraisal of an induced arousal state determines the name humans ascribe to a feeling state. Thus, whether one feels angry, sad, fearful, or happy depends to a large extent on one's cognitive appraisal of these perceived changes in arousal. Lazarus's (1977) work also suggests that only those perceptions that have "emotional" meaning effect change or are "attended to."

These considerations have two important corollaries for the rehabilitation neuropsychologist. First, disturbances in brain-stem and related structures may influence basic arousal and/or attentional mechanisms. As such, goal-seeking (motivational behaviors) and the interruption of ongoing behaviors for biological-social (emotional) reasons may be altered because basic arousal and attentional dimensions of behavior have been impaired. In severe cases, unless this can be altered by medication and/or environmental stimuli, little can be done to help the patient learn and socially adapt. Even months or years after traumatic brain injury, some patients' "personality" difficulties may be secondary to brain arousal and attentional deficits.

Second, disturbances of higher "cerebral" or "cortical" centers may influence the ability of the person to perceive and interpret correctly feelings in self and in others. These emotional and motivational disturbances flow not from a lack of sustained or modulated arousal but from an inability to deal cognitively with arousal-producing stimuli. Therapies aimed at the cognitive underpinnings of these types of personality disturbances are vital. Conversely, in cases where there is diffuse cerebral dysfunction and associated impairment in abstract reasoning skills (see Luria 1966), traditional forms of psychotherapy or the so-called cognitive behavior therapies may be relatively ineffective. In cases of localized cerebral injury, however, or where abstract reasoning and memory skills are greatly preserved, such therapies may be quite effective and desperately needed by certain patients.

A consistently demonstrated finding in the animal literature has been that general visceral regulation and control of feelings are performed by highly complicated and differentiated mechanisms of the hypothalamus and the amygdaloid complex. Pribram (1971) reviewed available evidence that the amygdala, with its ventral medial hypothalamic connections, seems to play a key role in "emotional feeling" states. Damage to the amygdala in animals by surgical intervention or electrical stimulation fails to influence basic appetitive behaviors once they start. Thus, disturbances due to failures to stop eating, fighting, or engaging in sexual activities for biological survival have been noted. Moreover, in humans who have had unilateral surgical removal of the amygdala, hypothalamus, and part of the temporal lobe, there is some evidence of a dissociation between subjective reported feeling states and publicly observable appetitive behavior (see Pribram 1971).

Amygdaloid monkeys also show disruption of their basic visceral, autonomic functioning as measured by habituation studies (see Pribram and Luria 1973; Pribram and McGuinness 1975). Some patients given stereotactic amygdalotomies show reduced rage reactions even when there is a history of severe aggressive behavior. One can indirectly surmise that the intact amygdala may be very important in the normal stop or interrupt functions of appetitive or emotional behavior (see Pribram 1971 for a detailed description).

Pribram (1971, 1977) also suggested that the basal ganglia and the connecting fiber tracts to the far lateral hypothalamic region play an important role in motivation. Neurochemically, this far lateral region appears to be replete with nigral striatal fibers that carry dopaminergic substances. These substances seem to be important for carrying out complex animated movements and performing what we often describe as purposeful or motivated behaviors. Thus, damage to the limbic system and basal ganglia may lead to very significant disturbances in motivation. This is especially important because lesions to these areas are common following traumatic head injury (Graham et al. 1978), as noted in the Introduction and in Chapter 1.

Given the importance of emotion and motivation for survival, the role that cognition plays in interpreting feeling states, and the variable learning histories, it is unlikely that a specific brain lesion will produce a specific personality deficit. However, different lesions may influence the neurophysiological substrates of emotion and motivation in predictable ways. This is in keeping with Luria's concept of functional systems and interrelated subsystems that underlie all adaptive complex behaviors. Valenstein and Heilman (1979) reviewed in some detail various affective disturbances associated with lesions of the central nervous system. Sackheim et al. (1982) and Bear (1983) reviewed the literature on hemispheric asymmetry and the expression of emotions. The reader is referred to those sources for a comprehensive review of this topic.

Common Personality Disturbances after Brain Injury

Common personality traits associated with brain injury often include being irritable, being impulsive, acting in socially inappropriate ways, being unaware of one's personal impact on others, being less motivated, and being more emotional. The emotional problems typically include poorer tolerance for frustration, greater dependence on others, insensitivity to others, and generally a more demanding attitude (e.g., increased helplessness). A scheme for classifying these and other common personality changes after brain injury has not yet appeared. However, Goldstein (1942) suggested that many of these problems may flow directly from the cognitive confusion (e.g., loss of abstract attitude) and increased fatigability commonly found in brain-injured patients. Some personality changes after brain injury truly reflect the struggle of the damaged organism to adapt to an environment that no longer takes into consideration limited cognitive skills and physical disabilities.

While some clinicians are impressed with the notion that the premorbid personality influences postmorbid personality changes (e.g., Schilder 1934), it is difficult to demonstrate this empirically. Kozol (1945, 1946), for example, was unable to show that pretrauma personality characteristics correlated with posttrauma "neurotic" symptomatology. Despite premorbid functioning, most trauma patients were described as "irritable" and easily frustrated following injury. These data and others suggest that affective disturbances after brain injury may be greatly influenced by the type and extent of neural damage. Yet in cases of particularly mild head injury, preexisting psychiatric disturbances may be correlated with later presence of general psychiatric disturbance. McLean et al. (1983) found no significant differences between closed-head-injury patients and peer groups (i.e., friends or matched relatives of the patients) on psychiatric symptomatology, and they suggested that others found psychiatric differences between groups because they used inadequate (cross-sectional) control groups (Weddell et al. 1980). Their study provides indirect evidence that closed-head-injury patients do not represent a typical cross-section of the population but may be more representative of people who were previously maladjusted or risk-takers. To some degree, this has been documented in children (Brown et al. 1981).

In more severe brain injuries, the role of the preexisting personality for postinjury personality disorders may be considerably lessened. For example, there is strong evidence that the severity of the brain injury is directly related to certain, but not all, psychiatric or behavioral disorders (e.g., Lishman 1968 and 1973; Levin and Grossman 1978; Levin et al. 1979).

Research on personality disturbances following brain injury, particularly traumatic head injury, suggests four broad "classes" of behavioral phenomena that seem especially important for neuropsychological rehabilitation: (1) anxiety and the catastrophic reaction; (2) denial of illness, or anosognosia; (3) paranoia and psychomotor agitation; and (4) depression, social withdrawal, and the so-called amotivational states. While some of these phenomena may occur more frequently with right-brain injuries than with left-brain injuries (e.g., anosognosia) or with temporal lobe dysfunction (e.g., paranoid ideation), they are so common in brain-damaged patients that they will be discussed without extensive detailed reference to possible neuroanatomical correlates.

ANXIETY AND THE CATASTROPHIC REACTION

"A patient may look animated, calm, in a good mood, well-poised, collected and cooperative when he is confronted with tasks he can fulfill; the same patient may appear dazed, become agitated, change color, start to fumble, become unfriendly, evasive and even aggressive when he is not able to fulfill the task. His overt behavior appears very much the same as a person in the state of anxiety, and I have called the state of the patient in the situation of success, *ordered condition*; the state in the situation of failure, *disordered* or *catastrophic condition*" (Goldstein 1952: 255). Goldstein (1942, 1952) eloquently described the plight of brain-injured adults and provided classical insights into why they may appear so emotionally labile. Unable to deal with their cognitive confusion (or decreased abstract reasoning skills), brain-injured patients can be easily threatened and experience an associated anxiety about life. Goldstein (1952) pointed out that many brain-injured patients have a strong need to discharge this tension or anxiety and frequently do so without the social amenities. This results in their being described as impulsive, as behaving inappropriately, and as psychologically unsophisticated. He pointed out that these patients experience a release of tension by such actions but do not necessarily feel a sense of enjoyment or freedom over their actions. Consequently, they are in a situation in which impulsive or inappropriate responses have a reinforcing quality (i.e., reduction of tension) but also bring punitive social reactions from the environment. This may simply add to the patient's confusion and feelings of hopelessness.

Studies that have assessed anxiety after brain injury typically do not report a strong relationship between the degree of anxiety and the degree of brain damage. Lishman (1968) investigated the relationship between psychiatric disability and indices of brain damage. Anxiety was not particularly related to estimates of posttraumatic amnesia or the degree of brain tissue destroyed. In contrast, signs of intellectual and memory impairment were related to these measures. Levin and Grossman (1978) reported a statistical relationship between the grade of the head injury and anxiety, but again the relationship was not clinically impressive. Prigatano (1983b) (as described in Chapter 2) classified forty-eight consecutive head-injury patients as "restless" or "not restless," based on their relatives' ratings on the Katz-R Adjustment Scale. Patients did not differ in age, education, length of coma, or chronicity of injury, yet the restless patients were described by relatives as notably more emotionally distressed. These data are in keeping with Goldstein's (1952) assertions that anxiety after brain injury may reflect the patient's struggle to adapt more than the degree or extent of brain injury and associated neuropsychological impairment.

Research on the catastrophic reaction has primarily been limited to whether the phenomenon is more common in patients with right-brain injury than those with left-brain injury. Gainotti (1972) compared patients with right versus left vascular and neoplastic lesions. On various emotional indices, left hemisphere patients were considered to show more signs of anxiety, tears, abusive language, and uncooperativeness. Yet there were no differences between the groups on aggressive behavior or depressive reactions. Also, some patients in each group showed all the signs of the catastrophic reaction. Gainotti (1972) further pointed out, however, that patients with Broca's aphasia were especially prone to show emotional outbursts. While this at first glance might be taken as a reflection of some specific relationship between anterior left hemisphere disturbance and the catastrophic reaction, a more parsimonious explanation is possible. These patients may have simply lost the linguistic and cognitive resources for dealing with their anxiety and consequently appear more emotional (see Dikmen and Reitan 1977). At this point, it appears that the catastrophic reaction is a common occurrence following brain injury and is associated with failures in coping rather than with a specific type of lesion.

The natural course of development of the catastrophic reaction over time is only starting to be investigated. Fordyce et al. (1983) reported that chronic head-injury patients frequently experience greater emotional distress than acute patients. This was based on self-report and on relatives' ratings of the patient's emotional and motivational behavior. These data suggest that with cumulative experiences of failure in the environment, patients can become more, not less, disturbed in their personality functioning. Prigatano (1981) reported that during the very early phases following brain injury, when cognitive confusion is perhaps greatest, the patient may experience relatively little emotional distress. During the first year following traumatic brain injury, however, the patient may become more emotionally distressed. At this time the patient tends to misjudge the degree of the cognitive deficit and attempts to return to work and social activities. The patient soon becomes frustrated and unable to cope. Family members typically see the patient as more belligerent, negativistic, and generally using poor judgment. After failing in the environment, the patient then tends to withdraw and generally becomes more suspicious of others. The catastrophic reaction may change its form as the patient's cognitive confusion lessens and the degree of contact with the environment changes. One coping strategy for many brain-injured patients may be simply to withdraw from the environment after repeated failures in dealing with it. Neuropsychological rehabilitation needs to address directly the problem of social withdrawal and interpersonal isolation following brain injury.

DENIAL OF ILLNESS, OR ANOSOGNOSIA

The phenomenon of frank denial of a neurological deficit or disease has been recognized for many years. Weinstein and Kahn (1955) provided a comprehensive overview of this phenomenon, as well as a method of classifying the types of denial that are clinically seen. They noted that the phenomenon is more frequent with nondominant (usually right) hemispheric lesions and is associated with alterations in mood, disorientation as to time and place, and/or nonaphasic misnaming errors. Patients with a right hemisphere cardiovascular accident and left hemiplegia can demonstrate striking examples of this phenomenon, particularly during the acute phase of their neurological illness. When asked to move both arms, for example, the patient may move only the right hand and say that the left is either "tired" or not wanting to move. If asked whether the left hand can move, the patient may state that it can and persist with this misbelief despite evidence to the contrary. As the acute period passes, this denial phenomenon may diminish or even disappear. Yet in many traumatic-head-injury patients with bilateral and deep brain lesions, denial of the severity of residual neuropsychological deficits may persist for many years posttrauma.

An interesting clinical example demonstrates the denial phenomenon and connects it with the catastrophic reaction. A twenty-three-year-old severe head-injury patient who remained grossly amnestic with cognitive confusion fourteen months after traumatic head injury was given a neuropsychological examination. The patient was asked if he had had any memory difficulties since his accident. He smiled and, in a very congenial manner, said no. The patient was then asked to listen and later recall the first story of the Logical Memory subtest of the Wechsler Memory Scale. After hearing the story, the patient tried to recall it but could give only one bit out of a possible twenty-two bits of information. He immediately swore at the examiner and the test, stated that he wanted the testing stopped, and would not participate in any form of rehabilitation. This behavior is found thousands of times in the course of neuropsychological evaluation of traumatic head-injury patients, although frequently in a less dramatic fashion. Such patients often insist that their residual neuropsychological deficits following head injury are mild or minimal, in contrast to relatives' reports that their deficits are significant and greatly disturb their day-to-day function. When confronted with this evidence, patients frequently become agitated and angry or withdraw.

This phenomenon suggests that denial is motivated by the need to keep out of awareness the harsh reality of cognitive, perceptual, and motor deficits. When these deficits are made obvious to the patient, the catastrophic reaction can and often does occur. Dealing with the problems of denial of illness and the catastrophic reaction is a major task of intensive neuropsychological rehabilitation. Unless these personality disturbances are dealt with, improvement in psychosocial adjustment seldom occurs. Awareness allows the individual to experience a normal grief reaction and to readjust to the lost skills and associated changes in body usage.

Research on the denial-of-illness phenomenon has centered on its frequency in right versus left hemisphere patients (Gainotti 1972). Its natural course is not well understood, nor are methods for dealing with it adequately outlined. Labaw's (1969) retrospective analysis of his own anosognosia following closed head injury is especially insightful. He reminded clinicians that, as a head-injury patient who had previously practiced as a physician, he was convinced that the impact of his brain injury was not that significant. Whether this reflects a psychological reaction to the painful realities of life following brain trauma (i.e., he was motivated not to recognize the threatening information about how he had changed), or true neurological disturbance in awareness and attention, needs to be evaluated more thoroughly in future research (see Heilman 1979). The work of Morrow et al. (1981) strongly suggests that disturbances of the right hemisphere may affect arousal level and consequently the capacity to respond to emotional stimuli. Their creative work suggests that the phenomenon of denial of illness may represent a neurophysiological disturbance as well as a psychological reaction to painful and emotional stimuli. Figure 3.1 shows that after right or left hemisphere brain injury there is a decrease in autonomic nervous system responsiveness to "emotional" stimuli. However, right hemisphere patients show less arousal to "emotional" and "nonemotional" stimuli. Thus, right hemisphere injury may specifically alter arousal and attentional mechanisms and thereby decrease the capacity for self-awareness.

In the clinical arena, it frequently appears that both neurological and psychological mechanisms are involved in the denial-of-illness phenomenon. For example, we have seen patients with primarily left hemisphere injury who have insisted that they have had no residual neuropsychological deficits despite repeated evidence to the contrary. In these patients, there is often evidence of premorbid problems in psychological functioning and social adaptation. Other patients seem to have fragmented cognitive and perceptual experiences and do not appreciate their deficits because of an organically mediated disturbance in self-perception. The interaction between the locus of the lesion, neuropsychological deficits, and the premorbid personality in producing various forms of denial of illness is worthy of further scientific exploration.

PARANOIA AND PSYCHOMOTOR AGITATION

During the acute period following traumatic head injury, many patients are restless, agitated, combative, and disoriented. They are easily confused and show signs of paranoid ideation. Antipsychotic medications are frequently administered to reduce psychomotor agitation. Many of these drugs seem to block postsynaptic dopamine receptors in the brain. In contrast, amphetamines are assumed to release dopamine and can, at high dosages, produce a similar series of behaviors known as amphetamine psychosis (Lipton et al. 1978). It appears, therefore, that either increases in dopamine or supersensitivity to dopamine immediately after traumatic brain injury may cause psychomotor agitation and associated cognitive confusion. One case report even suggests that dextroamphetamine may decrease confusion and paranoia following craniocerebral trauma (Lipper and Tuchman 1976). Theoretically, this alters dopamine levels in the brain.

Case reports with schizophrenic patients indicate that neuroleptic medications can exacerbate psychotic symptoms in some patients. It has been suggested that increases of plasma levels of haloperidol (one antipsychotic medication known to increase dopamine levels) account for this paradoxical effect (Tornatore et al. 1981). We have seen two traumatic head-injury patients who, on receiving haloperidol, showed increased restlessness, agitation, and paranoid ideation. Stopping the medication resulted in reducing these symptoms greatly. Apparently, obtaining the right balance of dopamine and related neurotransmitters after traumatic head injury may be necessary to reduce psychomotor agitation and paranoid thinking.

Several weeks or months after the acute phase of trauma, some patients continue to be restless and have thought disorders similar to functional psychosis. Schilder (1934) was one of the first clinicians to note this. Later, Lishman (1968) cited earlier work that suggested a special frequency of "schizophreniform" psychosis associated with left temporal lobe disorder. He also cited work that linked violent behavior to lesions of the medial temporal lobe. Damage to this region frequently includes impairment of the amygdala. As the earlier discussion indicated, such damage may produce problems in controlling the appetitive behaviors, particularly fighting.

Convex and inferior temporal lobe structures are known to be important for visual discrimination (Pribram 1971). It is quite possible that lesions to this region interfere with the interpretation of visual inputs from the environment; this could enhance or mediate paranoid interpretations of the

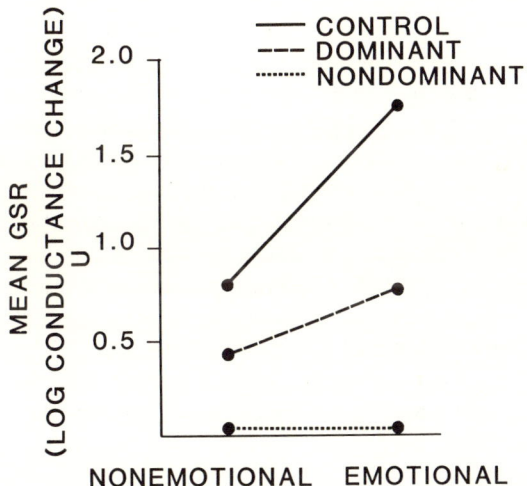

Figure 3.1. Galvanic Skin Response (GSR) to Emotional and Nonemotional Stimuli in Patients with Dominant and Nondominant Hemispheric Lesions. Reprinted, by permission, from Morrow et al. 1981.

world. Ferguson et al. (1969), for example, found notable paranoid tendencies in the interpretation of visual cartoons by temporal lobe epileptic patients. Thus, paranoid ideation, in some brain-injured patients, may flow from neuropsychologically based perceptual and cognitive disturbances. Leftoff (1983) provided a case study that argues that paranoia after brain damage is linked to disordered cognition.

Preexisting personality difficulties also appear to contribute to paranoid ideation. It is reasonably well accepted psychiatric principle that failure to establish basic trust and confidence in parental figures during early childhood is commonly found in paranoid individuals (Freedman et al. 1976: 489). For example, one closed-head-injury patient with severe memory disorder (Memory Quotient = 76 over five years, postinjury) insisted that others did not talk to her, actively avoided her, and despised her. This was contrary to overwhelming evidence that relatives and friends were willing to work and live with her despite her paranoid tendencies and memory disturbance. This patient's history, as corroborated by relatives, suggested that early in life she had developed a strong feeling of unworthiness and associated self-hatred. Before her accident, she was able to compensate for these problems by keeping socially active and doing good deeds for others. After the accident, she was unable to carry out her social activities, and this seemed to precipitate the development of paranoid ideation, which did not decline as her cognitive functioning improved. Another patient who had equally poor memory but no premorbid history of distrust in the environment showed none of these paranoid ideations.

Frank paranoid ideation and psychomotor agitation are extremely complex phenomena and may reflect disturbances in neurotransmitters and alterations in the perceptual and cognitive systems following neural damage, as well as be related to preexisting personality difficulties. Treatment of this class of behavioral problem requires a team approach. The patient should be tried on psychopharmacological medications, undergo a thorough neuropsychological analysis to see how perceptual and cognitive impairments may influence paranoid ideation, and be treated by an experienced psychotherapeutic clinician aware of how early childhood experiences influence later (paranoid) perceptions of the world. This class of personality disturbance appears to be one of the most difficult problems to treat after brain injury and makes psychosocial adjustment an impossibility if not substantially modified.

DEPRESSION, SOCIAL WITHDRAWAL, AND AMOTIVATIONAL STATES

The fourth class of personality disturbance seen after acquired brain injury in adults is a mixture of affective problems that results in an apparent lack of commitment to the rehabilitation process by the patient. While caused by different factors, three clinically identifiable problems can be classified under this dimension: depression, social withdrawal, and the so-called amotivational states.

Depression covers a broad scope of affective disorders (Freedman et al. 1976). As applied to patients who have suffered damage to the brain, it typically includes feelings of worthlessness, helplessness, guilt, loss of interest in work and family activities, and decreased libido. It also includes a sense of catastrophic loss over abilities which at times truly immobilizes the individual. It can be distinguished from normal sadness over the loss of cerebral function, social status, and employment. Sadness over a loss of function is a normal response to bad news. When patients receive good news, as reflected by improvement in their function, increased social acceptance, and so on, the sadness typically lessens if not disappears. In depression, such good news is met with no shift in the affective state. The patient appears to hang onto the cognitive structures that perpetuate feeling bad, feeling helpless, and maintaining a nonproductive approach to life. Depression is extremely common after brain injury, but does not seem to be especially related to the actual severity of the brain injury (Lishman 1968; Levin and Grossman 1978) or to the level of neuropsychological impairment (Prigatano 1983*b*). It also appears to be as common in right hemisphere patients as in left (Gainotti 1972). However, in patients who have frank denial of illness, which is more frequently associated with nondominant hemisphere injury, depression is less common. Depression is also more common in acute left hemisphere stroke patients (see Finkelstein 1982). Earlier psychometric studies have shown that depression is the single most common affective complaint of brain-injured patients several months after the injury, as measured by the MMPI (Reitan 1952).

Social withdrawal, which may be a part of a depressive syndrome, can also exist when no depression is present. After repeated failures in coping with the environment, many brain-injured patients simply withdraw to a safer milieu. This typically includes less social contact with others. The degree of social withdrawal has been related to the severity of the injury (Levin and Grossman 1978) and residual neuropsychological impairment (Prigatano 1983*b*). Unlike depression, therefore, social withdrawal may be indirectly related to the severity of brain dysfunction and consequent failures in coping with the environment.

As the discussion on catastrophic reaction suggested, many brain-injured patients initially do not expect to meet with as much failure in the environment as they do. Once they become aware of their failures, social withdrawal may be part of their natural tendencies to avoid anxiety and the catastrophic situations. Working with patients in a group can be of great help in dealing with the problem of social withdrawal and isolation, since such group work by its nature reduces social isolation and places the patients in an environment in which they can more easily relate and cope. However, group work does not necessarily help depression. In order for psychotherapeutic work to change depression substantially, it is necessary to change the patient's cognitions about self, either by group methods or individual methods. The depressed patient can remain depressed even though his or her social isolation is reduced.

Finally, there exist the so-called amotivational states that are frequently attributed to bilateral frontal lobe dysfunction. Benson et al. (1981) described schizophrenic patients who received prefrontal leucotomies and showed severe apathy several years postoperation. Yet, as they note, this affective problem was common even in the nonoperated schizophrenics. In his excellent analysis of frontal lobe function, Fuster (1980) described patients with severe frontal lobe pathology as lacking perspective with respect to past and future events. This cognitive deficit, coupled with the well-known disorders of attention manifested by easy distractibility, helps explain why frontal lobe patients often appear amotivational. It is hard for these patients to develop a plan of action (i.e., to be motivated) and to follow through on such a plan because of difficulties in sustaining attention. Information-processing theories (Simon 1967) and the basic model of emotional and motivational disturbances presented earlier would suggest that such amotivational states may in fact be a result of cognitive difficulties and not a disturbance in basic feeling states per se. A case example highlights this point.

A young adult traumatic head-injury patient with bilateral frontal lobe injury was noted to be very slow in his thinking and actions. It was assumed that he had a paucity of feelings and decreased drive state. The patient was involved in intensive neuropsychological rehabilitation for one year. During that time, he reported having feelings but often would report them in a slow and easily distractible manner. When this patient was given a plan of action by others (as opposed to being asked to generate the plan himself), he proved to be one of the most motivated patients. Given external structure, he would practice on tasks repetitively, often fatiguing those involved in his care. He worked diligently and was eventually able to become employed, albeit in a sheltered setting. This patient's performance raises the question of whether the amotivational symptomatology associated with frontal lobes is truly a problem of reduced drive, or a secondary problem related to cognitive (i.e., planning) difficulties. This case also demonstrates the dissociation of reported feelings (by the patient) from actual behavior. Slow, easily distracted patients may not be unmotivated; they are often just confused.

In summary, problems encountered by the rehabilitation neuropsychologist which seem to undercut the patient's commitment or drive to work at rehabilitation are frequently reflections of depression, social withdrawal as an attempt to avoid the catastrophic condition, and inability to generate a plan of action (so-called amotivational states). These problems can be separated from one another — and in fact must be, in order to develop an appropriate treatment plan.

Personality Disturbances in Brain-injured Children

Developmental changes of the central nervous system during the prenatal and early postnatal period are exceedingly rapid and complex (Curtis et al. 1972). Injury to the brain during this period is known to carry severe consequences for intellectual development in some children (Woods 1980). Injuries during the fifth to fourteenth years also have definite effects on problem-solving ability and memory and are related to the severity of the brain injury (Chadwick et al. 1981; Rutter 1981). But what impact do early cortical and subcortical lesions have on personality development? This question has been extremely difficult to answer for a number of reasons, which Rutter (1981) has reviewed.

In clinical practice, one is often impressed with parents who insist that their child's behavior was normal, if not above average, prior to the brain injury. They can list in exquisite detail a myriad of behavioral problems that the child has had postinjury. This point of view was eloquently described by Taylor (1959) in describing the personality of a boy who suffered a severe head injury at age seven. The work of Rutter and colleagues, however, suggests a different story (Rutter et al. 1980; Chadwick et al. 1981; Brown et al. 1981; Rutter 1981). In reviewing their work Rutter (1981: 1539–40) stated:

> Findings were striking in showing a strong relationship between the children's preinjury behavior and their psychiatric state at the one year follow-up. Of the children with no behavior difficulties before the accident, half were psychiatrically normal one year later, whereas this was so for none of those who showed mild behavioral problems before the head injury. Preinjury behavior was a strong predictor of children's psychiatric problems after severe head injury.

These data suggest that the incidence of new psychiatric disturbances after brain injury may be high (i.e., 50 percent) but that preexisting behavioral disturbance plus acquired brain injury ensure subsequent behavioral problems. It is important to document, from more than one source, the child's behavioral characteristics prior to the injury in order to evaluate emotional and motivational problems postinjury. Behavioral scales such as the Child

Behavioral Checklist (Achenbach and Edelbrock 1981) may be especially helpful in this regard.

The personality problems of brain-injured children are often classified under the rubric of social inappropriateness (see Rutter 1981; Brown et al. 1981). The child often says embarrassing things, reflecting poor judgment of the social situation. In addition, the child may be overly talkative, impulsive, careless in dress or manner, and forgetful of school and social responsibilities. It is interesting to note that impulsivity and hyperactivity were not considered by Rutter and colleagues to be the *sine qua non* of brain damage. Also, such problems as lying and stealing were as common in orthopedic control patients as in brain-injured patients (Brown et al. 1981). The same could be said for general responses to affective distress, such as nail-biting, enuresis, and phobias.

The family situation appears to influence these behavioral problems greatly. Rutter's more recent work, as well as that of Shaffer et al. (1975), suggested that adverse social and family situations increased the likelihood of psychiatric disturbance in brain-injured children. In fact, a measure of psychosocial disadvantage correlated more with psychiatric disturbance in brain-injured children than the extent of coma. It appears that brain-injured children, like adults, show symptoms that are as much a function of the environment as they are a function of neural damage. This must be kept in mind when evaluating and treating such patients.

The emotional and motivational disturbances in brain-injured children have generally received little attention. Such problems have been reported to be frequent in children with supratentorial lesions or cranial irradiation (Kun et al. 1983). Periodic clinical reports suggest that hydrocephalic children may be hyperverbal and uninhibited (see Prigatano and Zeiner, in press), but there are no systematic studies that look at the type and locus of brain pathology and the different environmental conditions that interact to produce emotional and motivational disturbances during childhood and their subsequent effect on personality development.

A Schema for Classifying Personality Disorders

Based on the above analysis and clinical experience, it has been useful to classify personality disorders after brain injury in adults and children along three broad categories. Some disturbances can be considered reactionary in nature, others are neuropsychologically based, and others are characterological or premorbid in nature. It may be helpful to the clinician to recognize that psychotherapy after brain injury might particularly address the reactionary problems, because they are generally not directly related to the degree of neuropathological changes or the resultant cognitive disturbances and instead simply reflect the overall difficulties the organism has in coping with the environment given limited adaptive skills.

The cognitive retraining activities, on the other hand, might address certain neuropsychologically mediated personality disorders. By focusing on the perceptual and cognitive difficulties, one may be able to undercut or at least reduce some of the neuropsychologically mediated disturbances in personality. The long-term or characterological problems may not be substantially changed by neuropsychologically oriented rehabilitation activities. Rather, simply engineering the interpersonal and work environment may be the best that can be done to help absorb or at least tolerate the long-term personality difficulties that a patient brings to rehabilitation.

While there is clearly no definitive list of the reactionary, neuropsychologically based, or characterological problems, the following are frequently seen in clinical settings as being typical for these broad categories.

Typical Reactionary Problems

Anxiety
Depression
Irritability
Mistrust of others
Hopelessness
Helplessness (i.e., more demanding attitude)
Anger
Social withdrawal
Phobias

Typical Neuropsychologically Mediated Problems

Impulsiveness
Socially inappropriate comments or actions
Emotional lability (includes poor tolerance of frustration)
Agitation
Paranoia
Unawareness of deficit (or severity)
Childlike behavior (giddiness or insensitivity to others)
Misperception of the intentions or actions of others
Apparent lack of motivation
Hypoarousal

Typical Characterological Styles

Obsessive or superorderly behavior
Hardworking attitude
Congeniality and friendliness
Social deceptiveness (psychopathic tendencies)
Desire to maintain satisfying interpersonal relations
Encouragement or discouragement of family support
Distrustfulness

Feeling not getting "enough" help from others and therapists
Avoidance of insight into self or discussion of personal topics
Enjoyment of upsetting others
Enjoyment of a dependent role
Defiant attitude (challenging therapist to go ahead and treat them if they can)

These lists are given to provide hypotheses that can guide clinical work. For example, when a clinician is faced with a patient who is very anxious or depressed or even irritable, it might be useful at least to begin with the notion that these are reactionary problems and could be addressed within the context of psychotherapy. In contrast, patients who are inappropriate in their social comments, paranoid, or unaware of their deficits might be viewed as having a neuropsychological basis for these difficulties and consequently in need of having these problems addressed in some form of cognitive retraining. Finally, patients who lack satisfying interpersonal relationships because of long-term disharmony at home and work might be viewed as characterological problems that can best be handled by environmental engineering as opposed to psychotherapy or cognitive retraining. Certainly the clinician can change his or her conceptualization of the problems as more clinical data are available. However, these lists might provide useful starting points in beginning to conceptualize how one would go about dealing with these personality disorders.

Psychosocial Consequences

Brain-injured patients frequently describe themselves as out of step with the rest of the world. They are often confused as to why others are upset with them and progressively withdraw. Common psychosocial problems after brain injury include an inability to maintain gainful employment, loss of pretraumatic friendships and relationships, impaired sense of body image, reduced self-esteem, and enhanced dependency on family and welfare systems.

Papers on psychosocial outcome often fail to communicate the impact of brain injury on people's lives, although there are some exceptions (Lezak 1978). In this context, Jennett (1978) made an interesting comment when describing what he would do, as a neurosurgeon, if his son were to suffer a traumatic head injury. After attending to the medical and surgical considerations, he, his wife, and his son would need sound psychotherapeutic help in facing the frustrations and personal crises associated with coping with the problems produced by brain injury. This family need is frequently overlooked in studies on psychosocial outcome after brain injury.

Table 3.1 Model for Assessing Psychosocial Outcome after Brain Injury

	Goal	
Subset	To Work (Be Productive)	To Love (Maintain Interpersonal Relations)
Discomfort	Unhappy with job performance and needing to work long hours to keep up previous productivity levels; decreased loss of self-confidence and enjoyment in work	Unwillingness to attend gatherings, progressive social isolation and withdrawal from others
Bizarreness	Excessive note-taking, repetition of questions already asked co-workers	Inappropriate social comments to spouse or children in public
Inefficiency	Unable to be gainfully employed, too slow in carrying out work activities, needing more structured supervision than the job normally requires	Spouse having to manage most of the family affairs, children feeling very uncomfortable in the presence of a brain-injured parent and avoiding contact with him or her

Assessing the psychosocial consequences of brain injury must ultimately include external, community criteria (e.g., the ability to return to work or drive a car), as well as personal or subjective criteria (e.g., the quality of interpersonal relationships between a husband and wife, or the degree of stress experienced by the parent of a brain-injured child). In the course of intensive neuropsychological rehabilitation work with brain-injured young adults at Presbyterian Hospital, a simplified model of psychosocial adjustment has evolved.

When asked by one interviewer what it meant to be psychologically normal, Freud purportedly responded: to work and to love. Translated into the rehabilitation arena, this might be stated as the ability to be productive (which often, but not always, includes gainful employment) and the ability to maintain interpersonal relationships. Buss (1966) suggested three other dimensions as qualifiers to these two broad classes of outcome behavior: discomfort, bizarreness, and inefficiency. Table 3.1 presents a model for evaluating psychosocial outcome in both objective and subjective terms for these two broad classes of behavior and gives examples of types of behavior that would fall within each cell of the grid.

In assessing a patient's ability to "work," researchers have typically assessed the inefficiency dimension. For example, Bond (1975) inquired whether a patient was able to return to a previous job or had to return to a lower form of work or no work at all. Using these types of criteria, the present best estimates are that approximately one-third of severe head-injury patients who walk and talk return to gainful employment (Weddell et al. 1980; Gilchrist and Wilkinson 1979; Bruckner and Randle 1972).

Predictors of returning or not returning to work are numerous. Emotional lability and postpsychotic states are clearly related to reduced work capacity (Bruckner and Randle 1972), and so are memory deficits (Bruckner and Randle 1972; Weddell et al. 1980) and severe communication disorders (Dresser et al. 1973).

While often not reported, subjective discomfort on the part of the patient returning to a particular work setting is common. Patients who previously held high-level positions and who have localized cerebral deficits may return to the old position only to be greatly stressed by it. Frequently, these patients have relatively isolated neuropsychological deficits (e.g., a visual-spatial deficit or a modality-specific memory deficit) and have a difficult time performing efficiently. They become progressively upset and disillusioned. Many eventually take a lower level of employment or seek psychiatric consultation. Weddell et al. (1980) reported, for example, a significant correlation between residual memory disturbance and personality disturbance after brain injury.

On the other hand, an inexperienced neuropsychological clinician may inadvertently assume that a mild head-injury patient's complaints are purely psychiatric in nature. If the patient is given standard clinical psychological tests of intelligence, memory, and personality, specific neuropsychological deficits may not emerge. The patient may then be placed in long-term insight psychotherapy that is not needed and that may in fact serve to upset the patient more, because the subtle underlying neuropsychological deficits are not understood and dealt with.

The changes in interpersonal relationships are the most difficult to assess scientifically, but they are of major importance to the patient's family. Walker (1972) eloquently listed how wives described the personality changes in head-injured husbands which substantially interfered with the degree of comfort and efficiency in their relationships. In keeping with the problem of self-awareness after brain injury, many traumatic head-injury patients (and cardiovascular-accident patients, for that matter) describe their residual difficulties only in terms of such physical factors as weakness or problems in walking. In contrast, spouses describe *both* physical and mental changes following brain injury. Notably, wives described their husbands as quick-tempered, fearful, easily fatigued, showing loss of interest in life and family activities, and prone to "fits of anger." Several wives mentioned in letters that husbands were impotent but frequently failed to state this during clinical interviews for fear of hurting their spouse's feelings.

Thus, in terms of the degree of comfort in interpersonal relationships, most if not all families experienced increased disharmony in their relationship with the brain-injured relative. If the patient is not working or being productive at home, there is certainly an inefficiency (i.e., a lack of reciprocity) in the interpersonal relationships. Many family members cannot comprehend personality disturbances following brain injury and frequently avoid the patient or assume that he or she "isn't trying." Weddell et al. (1980) noted, for example, that personality changes after trauma resulted in a significant loss of preaccident friendships.

While family members can often tolerate a brain-injured young adult who cannot be gainfully employed, they have an extremely difficult time handling the breakdown of interpersonal relationships. Paranoid, depressed, and belligerent brain-injured patients put by far the most stress on family members. While the divorce statistics for head-injury patients versus non-head-injury patients are unknown, termination of the marriage or long-term separation from the spouse and family is common. Increased dependency on other family members and public welfare systems thus becomes a common psychosocial problem.

A final psychosocial outcome worthy of further investigation is the incidence of psychiatric illness in the spouse and children of brain-injured adults. While Rutter's (1980, 1981) works implicate the parents' psychiatric state as a precursor for mild head injury in children, that is only half the story. The problems of brain injury can enhance psychiatric distress in parents and spouse. For example, Mash and Johnston (1983) reported decreased self-esteem and enhanced stress levels in mothers of hyperactive children.

Summary

Disturbances in personality are common after acquired brain injury in adults and children. They are frequently overlooked because they lack diagnostic utility, but they are crucial for rehabilitation planning. Because there is no universally agreed on definition of personality, and because most theories of personality are not related to models of brain function, neuropsychologists have not systematically studied emotional and motivational problems after brain injury. Yet there are clusters of common personality disturbances after brain injury in adults which should be recognized, particularly by the clinical neuropsychologist involved in rehabilitation.

While it is unlikely that a specific (i.e., focal) brain lesion will produce a specific personality disturbance, different lesions may influence various neurophysiological and neuropsychological substrates of emotion and motivation in predictable manners. Some lesions will influence arousal and attentional mechanisms, others will influence the cognitive appraisal of feeling states and the manner in which feelings are expressed. Premorbid personality and present social situations also greatly influence the form of affective response after brain injury.

Personality disturbances after brain injury have been shown to influence psychosocial adjustment greatly. Work and interpersonal relationships cannot be adequately maintained unless these affective problems are modified. Methods of personality assessment and therapeutic intervention are greatly needed for the rehabilitation of brain-injured adults and children.

CHAPTER 4
Cognitive Retraining in Perspective

George P. Prigatano

The description of the cognitive and personality deficits in the preceding chapters leaves little doubt that these deficits contribute greatly to the psychosocial difficulties of brain-injured patients. If these disturbances could be reduced and improvement in basic higher cerebral functioning could be achieved, substantial benefits would accrue. The question is: Is cognitive remediation possible?

The answer is difficult to obtain because of the inherent problems in defining cognition and cognitive deficits and thereby in knowing how to approach them within a remedial or rehabilitation setting. It does appear that something can be done to improve higher cerebral functioning after brain injury and that consequently cognitive retraining should proceed more as an evolving hypothesis than a tried and true method of treatment. In fact, when placing cognitive retraining in perspective, many different ideas emerge regarding its use and definition.

There is presently great interest in remediation of cognitive deficits after brain injury. In fact, it is considered an important part of modern rehabilitation of the brain-injured patient (Rosenthal et al. 1983). While the terms *cognitive rehabilitation, cognitive remediation,* and *cognitive retraining* are relatively new, the underlying concepts and the phenomena they address have been well known for some time. In 1947, Oliver Zangwill, a noted British psychologist, eloquently described the issues and goals involved in cognitive retraining with brain-injured patients. A few years earlier, Kurt Goldstein (1942) emphasized the importance of cognitive (and personality) deficits associated with brain injury and outlined basic principles of what might today be called "cognitive" or at least neuropsychologically oriented rehabilitation. Luria published his famous work on the restoration of higher cortical function after brain injury in Russian in 1948. While English versions did not appear until the 1960s, his work was most influential because it suggested a neurological model for explaining total or partial recovery of function, something that had not been done by previous theorists.

Despite these past works and more recent efforts (see reviews by Darley 1972; Sarno 1976; Kertesz and McCabe 1977; Ben-Yishay and Diller 1983), the basic questions that Zangwill raised remain: "We wish to know, in particular, how far the brain-injured patient may be expected to compensate for his disabilities and the extent to which the injured human brain is capable of re-education" (1947: 62-63). What Zangwill wrote at that time is true today: "Alas, no categorical answer can be given."

Yet, since the 1940s, additional information has been obtained regarding the nature of cognitive deficits following various types of brain injury, particularly traumatic brain injury (Levin et al. 1982). In addition, the processes underlying the recovery of function have been more thoroughly investigated (Fingers 1978; Kertesz and McCabe 1977), and the efficacy of various forms of cognitive remediation has received some attention (see Gianutsos and Gianutsos 1979; Gasparrini and Satz 1979; Prigatano 1983a; Weinberg et al. 1977; Weinberg et al. 1982; Miller 1980). While systematic research on cognitive retraining is still lacking, there are enough data and clinical experience to put present-day cognitive remediation into perspective. By having an appreciation of the historical, clinical, and scientific basis of modern cognitive retraining, rehabilitation professionals may be able to avoid unrealistic expectations and plan the use of cognitive remediation procedures in a more systematic manner.

The Historical Perspective

Faced with the problems of rehabilitating soldiers from World War I and World War II, Goldstein (1942) was perhaps the first modern neurological clinician to consider seriously both the psychiatric and residual higher cerebral dysfunctions faced by brain-injured patients. His insights into the nature of mental symptoms following brain injury and the predictable catastrophic reaction that most brain-injured patients experience formed the cornerstone of psychologically oriented rehabilitation today. Goldstein (1942) recognized that three classes of symptoms could underlie the mental or neuropsychological disturbances of brain-injured patients. One group of symptoms were not a direct result of damage to the brain per se. Instead, they reflected the struggle of the organism, given its deficits, to cope in the environment. A second class of symptoms were those that reflected direct damage to specific areas of the nervous system. For example, aphasia, memory disorder, motor disturbance, and sensory problems could be tied to specific areas of brain dysfunction. A third class of symptoms were those that were a result of what Goldstein called the "impairment of the abstract attitude." These symptoms were less easily defined, but Goldstein felt that many of the "personality" problems of brain-injured patients really reflected this class of difficulties (see Chapter 3).

Goldstein was convinced that symptoms that reflect a struggle to adapt could be drastically helped by careful planning of the rehabilitation process. He recognized the need for psychological assessment of patients' deficits and urged moving patients progressively from a state of convalescence to productivity. If patients could work a few hours a day, they should be given a trial at real-life work activities outside the sheltered environment. One is hard-pressed to find a more elegant description of brain-injured patients' needs than Goldstein's 1942 work.

Shortly after Goldstein published his work, Zangwill (1947) presented his ideas concerning the issues faced by psychologists who attempt to rehabilitate brain-injured patients. In his paper entitled "Psychological Aspects of Rehabilitation in Cases of Brain Injury," he specifically raised the question of whether a damaged brain could substantially be taught to recover lost functional capacities. Many of his examples included work with aphasic patients, since language disorders were more commonly recognized at that time and were dealt with from a rehabilitation point of view. Zangwill was aware, however, that what he called "direct retraining" may have limited success in helping brain-injured patients actually regain lost higher cerebral functioning. As a consequence, he identified two other principles of reeducation or remediation: "compensation" and "substitution." "By compensation is meant broadly a reorganization of psychological function so as to minimize or circumvent a particular disability" (p. 63). He felt it was most important to emphasize that the nervous system naturally shows a method of compensation after a lesion has occurred to healthy cerebral tissue. He credited Hughlings Jackson (1835–1911) for pointing out that there are both positive and negative manifestations of reorganization in the brain following injury. Once a central nervous system lesion occurs, brain-injured patients attempt to compensate. Zangwill believed that the compensation for the most part was spontaneous in nature and occurred without the patient's explicit intention. He considered that psychologists (or any rehabilitation therapists) could potentially carry the patient's efforts at compensation further by direct instruction and guidance. He gave examples of doing this, particularly with patients who have various types of aphasic disturbances.

In addition to compensation, Zangwill (1947) felt that the phenomenon of substitution was very important. "Substitution may be defined as the building up of a new method of response to replace one damaged irreparably by a cerebral lesion" (p. 64). Thus, he felt that one form of remediation was to teach a person a new response method when a certain response could no longer be obtained. For example, teaching braille to the blind was one method of substitution training. In substitution the brain-injured patient is actually solving a problem that he or she is capable of solving, but using new methods of approaching the problem. This is a higher level of functioning since it is not having to avoid solving an old problem but rather finding new ways of going about solving that problem. Zangwill felt that many factors limited the degree to which the patient could use substitution. Certainly the degree of brain dysfunction, and particularly the presence of diffuse cerebral injuries versus circumscribed cerebral injuries, was considered an important variable. This observation that diffuse injury carries with it much more devastating effects for cognitive retraining was first recognized in print by Zangwill and later by other psychologists (see Newcombe 1969).

The highest order of training in which the brain-injured patient could be involved was direct retraining. Zangwill (1947) was cautious about whether direct retraining was possible, but he believed that it should be attempted in order to gain a body of information that would guide rehabilitation activities for various types of patients in the future. By working repeatedly to improve memory and/or thinking, some recuperation of a lost function might be possible.

These three principles — the use of compensation to get around a deficit, the use of substitution to solve a problem that the brain is able to solve, but by different methods, and finally, attempts to retrain specifically impaired functions directly — represent the three basic approaches to cognitive retraining that can be found today.

Luria's (1948) work emphasized some of the same principles, but he argued for the importance of directly intervening in the functioning of the nervous system to facilitate the rate of recovery. His ideas were revolutionary insofar as they suggested that the brain may be in a state of inhibition following the occurrence of a lesion. Psychopharmacological approaches should be used to "deinhibit" brain function in order to restore its higher-order capacities. The use of pharmacology coupled with teaching methods was the cornerstone of Luria's approach to rehabilitation. It is by far the most modern view that has been produced in the scientific literature. Still, no systematic body of research has tested Luria's revolutionary and heuristic concepts.

Luria et al. (1969) talked about the use of anticholinergic medications to restore the brain to a level of deinhibition that would facilitate the transmission of nerve impulses across synaptic clefts. He also felt that there was a role for what he called "pedagogic" deinhibitory therapy. By this, he meant simply that teaching methods could also be used to help the brain recover its functional capacity at a faster rate. Today we might say that certain forms of cognitive retraining might help reduce the patient's degree of confusion and increase his or her efficiency in processing information.

Luria et al. (1969) identified two broad forms of restoration of function as a result of this pedagogical intervention. One form was the apparent restoration of function by transfer to the opposite hemisphere of that function. This is the classic notion that, for example, restoration of language function after a left hemisphere lesion may be possible because the right hemisphere could "take over" that function. In Zangwill's terms, this seems to represent a form of substitution training. In addition to this type of restoration of function, however, Luria felt that a reorganization within a given brain-functional system or subsystem was possible. That is, while a certain area of brain damage may interfere with the ability to do math or arithmetic or any of the other higher-cortical functions, that area could be retrained to reorganize itself to carry on that function. In a sense, this is a higher-order level of reorganization within multiple levels of brain interaction. Luria essentially agreed that compensation training was also useful particularly for patients that had diffuse brain injury as opposed to focal lesions, but his English writings did not actively address this topic.

These historic ideas concerning retraining after brain injury have remained the cornerstone of modern-day cognitive rehabilitation. Few, if any, substantially new ideas followed the contributions of Goldstein, Zangwill, and Luria. In the 1950s and 1960s, greater emphasis was placed on defining the nature of the neuropsychological deficits associated with various brain injuries than on developing rehabilitation strategies. However, a change in emphasis occurred in the late 1960s and early 1970s. Papers by Darley (1972), Sarno (1976), and Kertesz and McCabe (1977) reviewed the work on recovery from aphasia and its treatment. Yet information on recovery from memory disorder, intellectual disturbance, and personality disturbances remained relatively sparse. It is only more recently that investigators have become interested in trying systematically to rehabilitate brain-injured patients into society.

A major breakthrough in the early 1970s prompted interest in this area. Yehuda Ben-Yishay and his colleagues at New York University greatly facilitated this change. Ben-Yishay had the task of rehabilitating soldiers injured in the Israeli wars. By developing an intensive milieu approach, he suggested that the potential level of social recovery may be greater than had previously been thought. Also, during the early 1970s at New York University, there was considerable research on the rehabilitation of stroke patients who suffered visual-spatial deficits as a result of right hemisphere lesions (Diller et al. 1974). These researchers and clinicians set the stage for the proliferation of interest and research on cognitive remediation.

Yet for cognitive retraining to continue to grow and expand, a new data base must emerge. The question is not only "Is the brain capable of reorganization and relearning after brain injury?" but also "How do you specify what kinds of functional abilities may recover with the passage of time?" and "What types of intervention influence the rate and eventual level of recovery?" It is important to note that cognitive remediation can be a useful adjunct to various forms of treatment if it simply helps the rate of recovery and does not influence the level. This would result in patients' being able to return to the home or to work at a faster rate than through traditional means. If cognitive remediation can also elevate the level of recovery, a substantial scientific as well as clinical breakthrough will occur. To this point, the evidence of this latter phenomenon's occurring remains questionable, but the quest should not be abandoned. The field is new, and research efforts should be directed at the efficacy of cognitive retraining as it influences both the rate and the level of functional capacity.

The Clinical Perspective

Faced with the practical problems of attempting cognitively to remediate or retrain a brain-damaged patient, what does one actually do? The answer is dependent on many variables, such as the severity of the brain injury and the resultant neuropsychological limitations, as well as the skill of the therapist. As general guidelines, however, the following points have proven to be clinically useful. First, the brain-injured patient may be more confused in his or her thinking than is obvious by direct examination. This is because neuropsychological testing, or any formal evaluation, is usually structured and patients do better in a structured situation than in a nonstructured one. Also, patients may have problems in day-to-day functioning which are not adequately assessed by formal diagnostic procedures. Thus, a patient may be able to learn a series of paired-associate words but be confused as to where the car is parked or what door to take to leave the office. Daily contact with severe closed-head-injury patients (and even those with localized brain injuries) makes it clear that the degree of cognitive confusion goes beyond what is typically suspected, even several years postinjury. Consequently, the first major goal of cognitive rehabilitation is to reduce the overall or generalized cognitive confusion.

Many different types of tasks can be used for this purpose, but the best tasks gently but systematically help the patients understand areas of difficulty. This is necessary so that patients can start to form some systematic conceptualization of their thinking, memory, judgment, and personality difficulties. This usually requires helping the patients improve in their attentional skills and gradually process information more efficiently (i.e., at faster rates).

Next, cognitive retraining should enhance the patient's awareness of his or her residual strengths as well as deficits. This allows the patient to see that not all abilities have been affected by the brain injury. It provides a source of realistic support and gives clues as to how the patient can compensate for residual and permanent neuropsychological deficits. This typically needs to be done in both individual and group settings, as will be described in Chapter 6.

Third, the patient must be helped to recognize the need for compensatory behaviors. There will be a natural resistance to this, because the use of compensations is a direct statement that one has suffered brain injury. For organic and/or psychiatric reasons, it is sometimes difficult for the patient to recognize this and to take steps to deal with the reality. Helping patients use compensatory behaviors often requires helping them come to grips emotionally with the reality that they have suffered a brain injury. The use of compensation techniques therefore presupposes that patients have come to a point where they can accept the effects of the brain injury on their life and take steps to deal with it realistically. Consequently, the third approach in any form of cognitive remediation must center on having the patients use compensatory techniques as they are helped to accept the consequences of their brain injuries.

The fourth step is to help the patients deal with their cognitive deficits not only in the presence of a given therapist but also as the deficits emerge in interpersonal behavior. As noted in the Introduction and in Chapter 1, the hallmark of effective cognitive retraining is not to treat a specific difficulty in isolation but to deal with that deficit as it impinges on a broader range of social behaviors. In most instances, families seek out cognitive retraining for a given patient not because he or she has a specific memory problem or perceptual motor difficulty but because these problems frequently make it much more difficult to live with the patient. Behind this is usually a broader set of cognitive and personality problems that cause the patient to behave in socially inappropriate ways and to be difficult to manage. Consequently, cognitive retraining must include dealing with the underlying cognitive and personality deficits of the patient as they emerge in social interaction.

These four steps are relatively simple in principle but may be difficult to put into practice. Chapter 6 will describe these basic ideas as they are used within the Neuropsychological Rehabilitation Program developed at Presbyterian Hospital. At this point, two clinical examples will be given to highlight the importance of these ideas. In the first case the four steps were applied and a reasonable outcome was obtained. In the second example, the four steps were not applied and the outcome was less favorable.

The first clinical example is that of a twenty-one-year-old single white male who suffered severe brain injury secondary to falling from a bridge. His CT scan revealed bilateral low-density changes in the frontal poles, involving the tips of the temporal lobes (see Fig. 4.1). Approximately one year postinjury, he had a WAIS Performance IQ of only 61, with an estimated Verbal IQ in the low 70s. He was extremely slow in his motoric

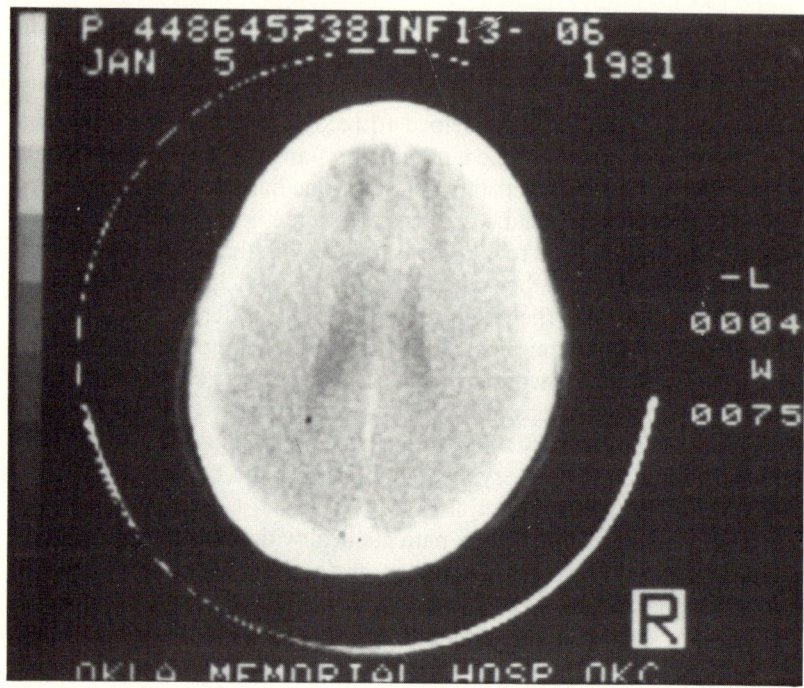

Figure 4.1. CT Scan Demonstrating Bilateral Frontal Atrophy in a Young Adult Male after Severe Craniocerebral Trauma. Courtesy of the Radiology Department, University of Oklahoma Health Sciences Center, Oklahoma City, Okla.

and cognitive functioning. His affect was flat, but he retained a sense of humor. He was unaware of the severity of his neuropsychological deficits and had very unrealistic occupational goals. For example, he initially said he wanted to be a short-order cook or a helicopter pilot.

Cognitive retraining began by having him carry out a series of simple psychomotor tasks that could be used to document his slow speed of performance. This gently helped him to recognize that he was much slower than the average person. The tasks also dealt with basic orientation materials so that he could reduce his general confusion and slowly become aware of his deficits as well as some strengths. Thus, the first two principles described were applied.

After the patient had plateaued in his psychomotor performance, he was taught different strategies for carrying out these simple psychomotor tasks that had not dawned on him. This resulted in some improvement in his overall speed of performance. Thus, he could see tangible evidence that using strategies (a form of compensation) might assist him when he no longer would expect any improvement. He was not lectured regarding the use of compensations; he could see firsthand their impact on his performance. However, despite the aggressive use of these strategies, he was not able to improve his overall level of psychomotor functioning substantially, even though some improvement did take place. For example, at the beginning of his cognitive retraining, his total time to complete the Trail Making Test, Part B, was 303 seconds. At the end of approximately six months of training, that score dropped to 201 seconds. While this was a substantial improvement, his level of speed was still considerably below average and made it impractical for him to be gainfully employed in any job that required normal psychomotor performance. The patient gradually recognized this through the help of his cognitive retraining exercises. He could literally plot his scores over several weeks and see what his rate of improvement was and, conversely, the amount of difficulty he had compared with other patients and to individuals who had not suffered brain injury.

This patient was also very slow when it came to responding verbally to others, so he was worked with in the context of cognitive group therapy (see Chapter 6), where he could receive feedback that his slow verbal responding was difficult on the listener. He consequently was taught to make compensatory statements to aid him in social interactions. For example, he might say, "I am thinking about your question, but it will take me a little while to respond." This allowed the listener to know what the patient was doing and not be put off by his slow thinking process. Thus, the compensation for severe psychomotor slowing was applied in a social context.

Principles three and four were therefore actively applied and used by this patient. He was treated not only individually for a cognitive deficit but also within a social milieu. In addition, he learned to compensate for these deficits in different ways, depending on the demands of the social situation. The compensations emerged slowly as he recognized the need for them and was able to accept the realities of his brain injury.

This patient eventually gave up his unrealistic occupational goals and began working in a sheltered workshop as a custodian. He was very impaired, and cognitive retraining may have only modestly changed his degree of cognitive dysfunction, but he is truly a rehabilitation success, due in part to cognitive retraining. He was able to show improvement in psychomotor functioning and was able to come to a greater awareness of his deficits. With this, he was able to accept these deficits and apply compensation techniques within the social setting. This allowed him to interact much more realistically with fellow patients as well as with others. Without this type of intervention, this man would simply have remained home and under the care of his parents.

This case also reaffirms the point that Zangwill (1947) suggested: for patients with severe bilateral cerebral dysfunction, the use of compensatory training might be more helpful than substitution retraining or direct re-

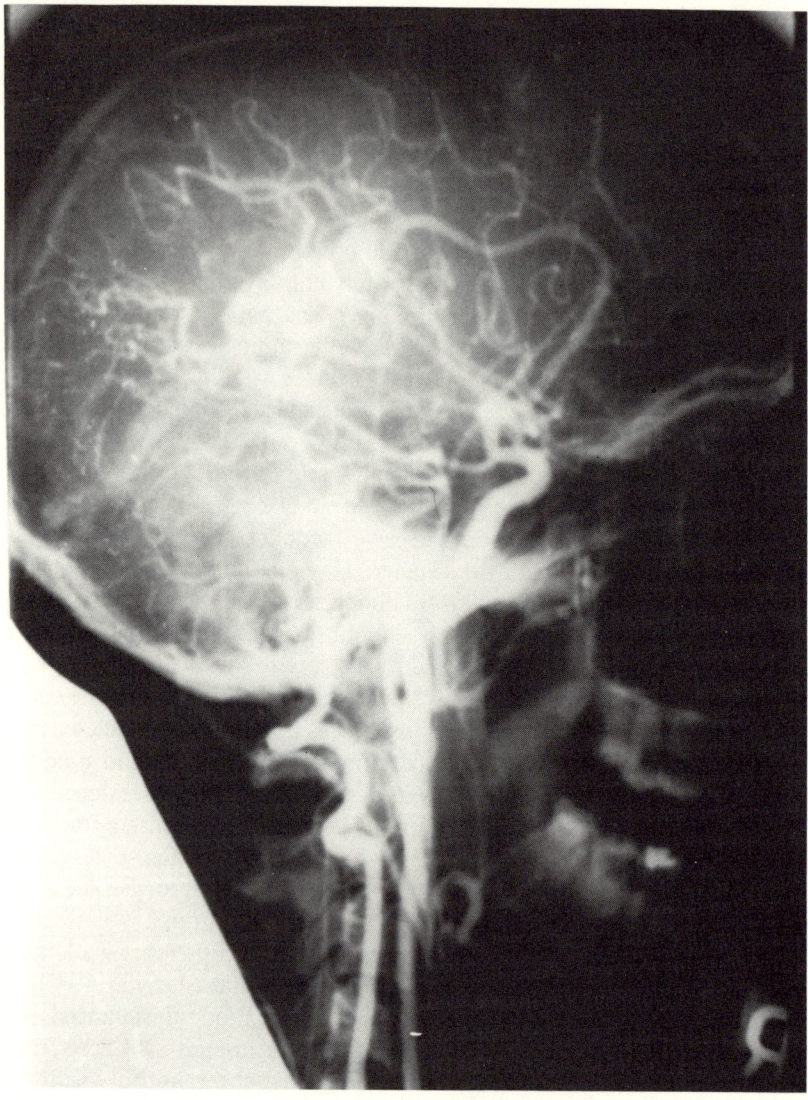

Figure 4.2. Cerebral Angiogram Revealing an Arteriovenous Malformation Involving the Corpus Callosum in a Young Adult Male before Surgical Removal. Courtesy of Charles Drake, M.D., London, Ontario, Canada.

training. Because many traumatically head-injured patients suffer this type of injury, the development of practical compensatory techniques is greatly needed, but little work has been done in this area. A fruitful area of cognitive remediation or retraining is the development of such compensatory techniques as they relate to memory difficulties, visual-spatial difficulties, attentional problems, and the variety of difficulties experienced under the category of "poor abstract reasoning."

A second clinical example is that of a young man with a localized brain injury, an apparently isolated cognitive deficit, who was treated *before* the four principles outlined above emerged as a result of clinical practice. At age twenty, this presently twenty-nine-year-old white married male suffered a subarachnoid hemorrhage. Neurological workup revealed a large arteriovenous malformation (AVM) that had invaded the posterior section of the corpus callosum (Fig. 4.2). The AVM was surgically removed, but in the process the splenium of the corpus callosum was sectioned. Right after the subarachnoid hemorrhage, the patient reported impaired memory skills, and six months following the surgical resection of his corpus callosum, complaints of a short-term memory deficit were still present. The neuropsychological examination at that time gave the impression that this man had suffered only an isolated difficulty. His IQ scores, as well as his performance on the Halstead Battery, were all within normal limits, but his Wechsler Memory Quotient was below average (MQ = 83). He complained that he could not remember names of people as well and had a difficult time keeping track of such things as important dates and appointments.

The patient was worked with initially from a limited cognitive retraining point of view. Because the neuropsychological examination gave the impression that visual-spatial skills were intact, he was taught basic visual-imagery techniques to aid his verbal recall (see Prigatano 1983*a* for details). The training lasted for approximately three months and seemed to aid his verbal recall substantially. For example, he was initially able to recall only 38 percent of the paired-associate words on the Wechsler Memory Scale, but after training he recalled 76 percent of these words. Six months posttraining, he recalled 72 percent of the words, so it was assumed that the cognitive remediation was successful, and the patient was discharged from treatment. Both he and his wife were grateful.

Approximately eight years later the patient returned. At that time, he stated that he had been depressed over his daily memory failures. He had been hesitant to return to see me because we had worked in cognitive retraining in the past and I believed that the treatment was a success and had even published a paper on it. He was embarrassed to come back and state that the treatment had not substantially helped him.

At first I thought that the patient was overstating his memory complaints. I readministered the Wechsler Memory Scale (Form II), paired-associated words, some eight years posttreatment. To my initial satisfaction, the patient was able to recall almost all the paired-associate words by the third trial. He had seemed to retain his basic visual-imagery skills. For example, when asked to remember the association "dig – guilty," he spontaneously said that he imagined the word "guilty" under the ground and that he was digging the word out. When asked to remember the association "necktie — cracker," he spontaneously stated that he imagined a tie wrapped around a large cracker. This resulted in his being able to retrieve most of the paired-associate words on psychometric tests. In the real world, however, he was never asked to remember paired-associate lists. He had to remember several bits of information at one time, and often those bits were not easily encoded using visual-imagery techniques. For example, he might have to remember previous work agreements, or where different employees were working and on what projects. Despite copious note-taking, he was exhausted by his memory failures. He tried to keep this a secret from his family and his employer. Only his wife knew of his memory difficulties, and she could not understand why he was so exacerbated by it. Even the patient wondered whether he was making up his problem or overexaggerating it. Thus, he had not become fully aware of the severity of the difficulty and its permanency despite the initial cognitive retraining. Furthermore, I had made the mistake of assuming that his problems in memory were actually isolated difficulties. Eight years later, I had him take a series of experimental cognitive tasks. One of them was the Shepherd Rotation Task, on which he demonstrated notable difficulty in visualizing mental rotations of geometric figures. None of this was observed on the formal initial psychometric assessment.

Thus, the first two principles noted above (i.e., recognizing that the patient may have more cognitive difficulties than are obvious, and helping the patient become aware of the deficits) were not adequately applied by the more limited approach to cognitive remediation. While the patient was willing to compensate for his difficulties, he had never really accepted his memory problems. He and certain family members felt that if he would only try harder his memory difficulties would improve. So the basic problem of acceptance of the deficit was not dealt with by the limited cognitive approach. Finally, the fourth principle of dealing with the deficit within the interpersonal setting was never adequately addressed, and this caused a major difficulty. He had hidden his deficits from his employer, and this was truly exhausting him and causing him great embarrassment. Only when he was able to go and tell the employer of his earlier surgery and his memory problems did he experience some relief in facing his problems. During an extended family session, this was discussed openly between him and his wife and other family members. It became obvious that while some could accept his difficulties, others could not. I believe that the failure initially to help this patient deal with this problem within the interpersonal context produced needless frustration during the eight years following his surgery. While there may be no ideal treatment, and while individuals will vary in their ability to benefit from the principles outlined above, it appears that deviating from these basic concepts is not helping the patient cope to maximum capacity with the problems that brain injury produces.

It is also of some interest that, even in this case of localized cerebral injury, the relative permanency of the neuropsychological deficit was made obvious by long-term follow-up. While the concept of plasticity of brain function is certainly inviting (Kinsbourne 1971), this particular case suggests that it may be overemphasized and that the basis of many forms of cognitive retraining may simply be to teach patients different strategies for dealing with their deficits (Gazzaniga 1978). This may consist of compensation training or substitution training, as described by Zangwill's earlier work. If this and other patients were worked with more acutely, perhaps one could demonstrate the effectiveness of direct retraining more adequately. At this point, however, these clinical examples lead one to suspect that the effectiveness of direct retraining is relatively sparse, at least in patients who are several months or years postinjury.

The two clinical case examples also highlight points that may be misleading to the cognitive retrainer. First, the initial neuropsychological assessment of patients does not automatically state how one should go about cognitively remediating deficits. There is a frequent misconception that the neuropsychological test findings will automatically suggest how to go about conducting cognitive retraining. In fact, this has never proven to be the case in my clinical experience. Rather, the neuropsychological test findings help clarify what areas of deficits and strengths exist in terms of an initial evaluation of a patient. However, only by living with the patient day-in and day-out does one really begin to understand a given patient's problems. In this context the development of retraining activities comes to mind. There are no series of tests (e.g., Luria's, Halstead's, Wechsler's) that automatically tell the clinician how to proceed in cognitive retraining. Such knowledge comes as a consequence of creativity and experience on the part of the clinician, as well as practical information about how brain injury affects different functional capacities.

The second point that these cases bring to light is that cognitive retraining, at least several months postinjury, may produce relatively little transfer or generalization effects. Diller (1976) raised this issue when he proposed a model for cognitive retraining and rehabilitation. Much of the research that Diller and his colleagues have subsequently done (e.g., Weinberg et al. 1977) focuses on this problem. It is extremely important and needs to be continually evaluated in clinical settings. Many times, brain-injured patients will learn specific behavioral strategies as they apply to specific environments but may not spontaneously generalize these behaviors to other environments. Consequently, if one wants to improve any area of cognitive dysfunction as it impinges on home or work life, it is vital that the cognitive retraining be done with family members and potential co-workers. It is not enough to try to deal with these behaviors in a rehabilitation setting and hope that they will generalize outside that setting.

Clearly, many clinical issues have to be kept in mind when attempting cognitive retraining. Considerable work is needed in order to develop systematic strategies for compensation as well as substitution and direct retraining when they seem to be appropriate. Research in this area must explore the effectiveness of the various types of interventions and provide a practical way to work with patients. Practicality implies not only easily applied methods of retraining but cost-efficient methods as well.

The Research Perspective

Research on cognitive retraining or remediation has centered on two broad methods of intervention. One dimension could be called the "milieu-based" programs, which attempt to resocialize brain-injured patients. The second has to do with specific cognitive remediation programs, or modules.

The milieu approach emphasizes more than cognitive retraining. Because its focus is on reintegrating the patient into society, it fosters not only the use of substitution training and direct retraining but also compensation training. Few reports have appeared in this area. Rosenbaum et al. (1978) reported on work with brain-injured patients in a milieu setting and emphasized that for some patients this seemed to be effective. However, there was no control group, and the degree to which various factors contributed to the patients' social reentry was undetermined. Ben-Yishay et al. (1982) provided a series of case examples demonstrating how various patients were able to return to gainful employment while others were not. Their clinical findings were supportive of the milieu approach, but no control group was utilized, nor were the guidelines for such training presented.

A controlled study on the milieu approach to working with brain-injured patients was reported by Prigatano et al. (1984) (see Chapter 7 for details). Eighteen traumatically brain-injured patients were compared with seventeen controls who were well matched on age, education, time since injury, and neuropsychological test characteristics. Modest improvement in neuropsychological test performance occurred in the patients who received the very intense milieu form of treatment. Also, the patients who received treatment showed substantial improvement in their affective functioning. It was surprising, however, that only 50 percent actually maintained gainful employment at the time of follow-up, compared with 36 percent for controls. This sobering fact made it clear that the milieu type of treatment program may help patients feel better about themselves, and in some instances actually improve neuropsychological test performance. However, the actual percentage of patients returning to work without a specific work trial was moderate. (This has broadened our perspective of what a milieu program should include and resulted in incorporation of a work trial as part of the rehabilitation program. See Appendix C.)

The milieu approach to cognitive retraining is important insofar as it brings to light all the variables that are important in the retraining of brain-injured patients. The problem of base rate recovery without this extensive form of rehabilitation, the question of whether the level of functioning is actually improved, and the rate of recovery of function require further scientific evaluation.

The research on specific remediational approaches has not been extensive, but data are available. An area of much interest has been memory retraining. At this time we have no therapies that make a poor memory good, but studies have tried to explore whether various types of mnemonic training would make a substantial difference. Gianutsos and Gianutsos (1979), using a single case design, showed modest improvement with repetitive practice. They attempted to teach patients ways of making words memorable, and this had a modest effect. Gasparrini and Satz (1979) specifically used visual-imagery training for patients with left cardiovascular accidents. They also reported modest improvement in verbal recall but clearly questioned the practicality of this form of treatment. Brooks (1983) recently reviewed a few reports on memory retraining and concluded that it is too early to evaluate its effectiveness. Recent books in the area (e.g., Wilson and Moffat 1984), however, emphasize "management of memory problems" versus remediation.

A second area of research interest has been perceptual retraining. Weinberg et al. (1977) demonstrated that right cardiovascular accident patients could be trained to improve substantially their ability to scan the left side of space. This resulted in improvement in the functional capacity to read. However, Weinberg et al. (1982) later pointed out that the assumed underlying cognitive process called "attention" or "perceptual scanning" was not substantially improved in nonneglecting right cardiovascular accident patients. Their data suggest that one can improve a specific functional capacity or skill (like reading) but not be able to improve substantially a basic underlying cognitive process when it is severely damaged. These data are in agreement with the notion that substitution retraining is helpful (as well as compensation training), but the effectiveness of direct retraining is doubtful, at least in this patient population.

A third area of research has been psychomotor retraining. Miller (1980) studied eight traumatic head-injury patients and four controls on a psychomotor task. The patients were asked to place various blocks into a form board. Subjects practiced daily, and learning curves were analyzed. It is not surprising that traumatic head-injury patients were slower in their learning and were not able to reach the same level of functioning as controls, but it is interesting that the rate of learning was also shown to be slower in these patients. The importance of practice or repetition as a method of compensation was emphasized by the authors.

These findings suggest that, at the present time, cognitive retraining has more to offer in the area of compensation and perhaps substitution than it does in direct retraining.

Summary

Present-day cognitive retraining ideas have been in existence for a long time. In fact, it is difficult to find any concept in cognitive retraining in the 1980s that did not exist in the 1940s. This is a humbling observation, but one that should be kept in mind.

At least three levels of cognitive retraining deserve clinical attention and research. The first is the practical goal of teaching brain-injured patients to compensate for deficits. In the cases of diffuse bilateral cerebral dysfunction, this may be the method of choice. The next level is to teach patients methods of substitution for solving problems. This involves using intact brain functions to get around the deficits to solve the same kind of problem. The third area is direct retraining, in which there may be an attempt to teach patients to improve an underlying functional deficit.

While there has been much interest in cognitive retraining over the last few years, many areas still need to be developed further if the field is to grow. Developing cognitive retraining methods to deal with the problems of unawareness and socially inappropriate behaviors is a broad area that needs intensive attention. In addition, it is necessary to develop cognitive retraining activities that take into consideration the role of personality variables so that the catastrophic reaction is not stimulated by such remediation.

CHAPTER 5
Psychotherapy after Brain Injury

George P. Prigatano

The psychosocial adjustment problems of brain-injured patients can frequently be substantially reduced. The preceding chapter focused on cognitive retraining as one set of activities aimed at helping the patient improve and/or adjust to residual neuropsychological sequelae of brain injury. It was emphasized that patients need to learn to become aware of their difficulties and learn to compensate for them when necessary. This requires a process of acceptance. Awareness and acceptance are never purely cognitive acts. Because they involve the affective side of life, psychotherapy is a vital component of any form of neuropsychologically oriented rehabilitation.

Psychotherapy is difficult to define because there are many schools of thought regarding the nature of human affective disturbances and how they should be therapeutically approached. A psychiatric consultant to our Neuropsychological Rehabilitation Program, Robert Wienecke, M.D., defines psychotherapy in terms of its broad outcome: teaching the patient (family and/or staff) how to learn to behave in his or her own best self-interest. This does not mean selfish interest; it means learning to get one's needs met in a fair and consistent manner. This definition, by nature, involves social value-judgments. What one considers to be in his or her best self-interest can vary in time and different social situations. We live in different social milieus and must either learn to adapt to all of them or change the environment to meet our needs, both biological and psychological.

A similar definition, which is couched in slightly different terms, comes from the Psychotherapy Research Project at the Menninger Foundation (Voth and Orth 1973). The effectiveness of psychotherapy (again defined by outcome) is measured in terms of the patient's ability to make "a deeper

---

An earlier version of this chapter was presented at the Models and Techniques of Cognitive Rehabilitation, Fourth International Symposium, Indianapolis, Indiana, March 31, 1984.

and richer commitment to life." This is typically defined as the enhanced ability to make honest and fair commitments to work and interpersonal relationships. Given their psychoanalytic approach, Voth and Orth (1973) offer an interesting description of how one measures the effectiveness of making these commitments: "Intrapsychic change can be assumed to have occurred if there is clear evidence that great commitment to life no longer triggers and activates unconscious conflicts. For example, if job promotions or marriage or children no longer evoke symptoms, one can assume that the core conflicts [typically] have been resolved to some extent" (p. 69).

Teaching brain-injured patients to make honest and fair commitments to life is possible, just as it is with non-brain-injured patients, and failure to do this may reflect the intrapsychic conflicts (as described by Voth and Orth 1973) or problems in learning and behavioral control secondary to brain injury or faulty pretrauma social learning (Ullmann and Krasner 1967). Clinicians who attempt to do psychotherapy with brain-injured patients need to realize that there are a great variety of possible causes for the emotional and motivational problems of the brain-injured patient. They should recognize that the process of psychotherapy with these individuals can be slow and more difficult because of the damaged brain (i.e., information-processing) systems. In other instances, the patient may be more open and less defensive because of frontal lobe injury. For the psychotherapist, the challenge of brain-injured patients is to determine how best to teach that brain or mind to do what can be done to alter either the environment or the patient's behavior in order to facilitate a fair and enhanced commitment to life. Of course, preexisting personality characteristics and the present family structure, as well as the degree and type of brain injury, will greatly influence this process.

The research on psychiatric illness following traumatic head injury is variable and in many instances nonsystematic, but the work of Rutter and colleagues (Rutter et al. 1980; Chadwick et al. 1981) has been enlightening. In their prospective studies a number of interesting facts come to light. First, the degree of psychiatric illness in head-injured children was related to the severity of the brain injury and the period of posttraumatic amnesia. However, a number of children who had mild head injuries had notable psychiatric disturbances if there were substantial indications of behavioral problems *before* the injury. Also, significant distress within the family was a clear predictor of behavioral problems in the mild head-injury group; in fact, in one study it predicted psychiatric status better than the length of the coma (Shaffer et al. 1975). These data make it quite clear that psychosocial as well as neurological factors contribute greatly to the psychiatric sequelae following brain injury.

Other researchers in the field have pointed out that brain-dysfunctional patients may show behavioral problems that are not directly related to the degree of neurological insult but have a profound influence on the patient's ability to function. For example, Levin and Grossman (1978) reported: "In an ongoing study of the neuropsychological, neurological, and social sequelae of closed head injury, we have been impressed with a distinct pattern of emotional and behavioral changes following injury and its contribution to prolonged functional disability, even in cases where there is no notable neurological or intellectual deficit" (p. 720).

Studying the neurological and psychological predictors of employability in epileptics, Dennerll et al. (1966) reported: "The results from this and other personality measures used in this project indicate that a general personality trait of *social competence or the ability to cope effectively with the interpersonal demands of different social situations* is an important factor in successful employment of persons with epilepsy" (p. 326; emphasis added). These observations make it quite clear that the rehabilitation-oriented clinician must address the personality disorders and psychiatric problems of traumatic head-injury patients if the clinician is to work realistically with them and return them to a productive life-style. Working with the families is inevitably an important part of this process (see Bond 1983). Effective intervention requires attention to the psychological needs of the people who live with and care for brain-injured patients (i.e., family and professional therapists) as well as the patients themselves. Thus, psychotherapy after brain injury must be directed first to the patient who has suffered the injury, but secondarily to those who must cope with the patient. This approach allows for a more reasonable management of the affective disturbances that are produced either directly or indirectly by brain injury.

Goals of Psychotherapy after Brain Injury

A hallmark of the live human brain that communicates with others is a search for understanding and then meaning. No matter how impaired a brain-injured patient is, he or she eventually asks the question "What has happened to me?" once consciousness is regained and the patient begins to become oriented. During periods of confusion the patient evokes a cognitive system to explain his or her perceptions (e.g., "I must be pregnant. Why else would I be in the hospital?"). The same brain that has lost part of the power of abstraction thus seeks out a cognitive explanation! Psychotherapy with brain-injured patients must start by providing an explanation. To do this, the psychotherapist must provide a model for understanding what has gone wrong that the brain-injured patient can handle. The model must be simple, but true as best the facts are known. It must make sense to the patient and be relatively easy to remember, while taking into consideration the major facts, scientific as well as personal. Finally, the explanation must explain much of what the patient experiences, irrespective of what he or she is able to verbalize.

The therapist must thus take on an active teaching role in the beginning. Knowledge of the neurological, neuropsychological, and psychiatric factors must be distilled and transmitted to the patient. This should be done not in a condescending manner but by streamlining the essential message. Patients do not need to be talked down to, no matter how impaired or confused they are. They must be treated as equals who have less capacity to understand the complexities of what is being said. Those who have successfully worked with mentally retarded adults make the same point (see Dean 1984).

As an explanation of what is wrong begins to unfold, there is usually the concomitant and more difficult question "*Why* has this happened to me?" The brain-damaged patient, just like the non-brain-damaged patient, wants to know and frequently provides his or her own answer. There is much self-blaming as well as blaming of others. Frequently, the patient sees the tragedy as a punishment for sins, or wants to punish others for causing the brain injury. This takes on many forms, but it boils down to the psychological reality that either "I was bad and deserve what happened to me" or "Others were bad and they deserve to be punished." Both alternatives must eventually be put aside so the patient can face the existential realities of life. This means that the patient must learn to live with the brain damage and still find meaning or commitment in life, which can be accomplished only when a good deal of self-acceptance and forgiveness have taken place. (This is the same for non-brain-injured psychotherapy patients.)

The process by which this is accomplished can be broadly described as the insight component. There is also clearly a need for behavioral management; that is, the patient must literally be taught new ways of behaving in order to maximize social competence. Insight alone or behavior management alone frequently does not cover the necessary steps in helping a brain-injured patient cope with personality disturbances.

Finally, it is my opinion that a third component is often necessary for psychotherapy with brain-injured patients. The psychotherapist and the rehabilitation team must instill a sense of hope in both the patient and the family. This sense of hope should not be blind, stupid, or naive, lest the patient think that he or she is indeed in incompetent hands. Rather, it should be realistic and reflect the human spirit to fight adversity and to overcome hopeless and helpless feelings. As we are fond of telling patients, we will try not to be overly optimistic or overly pessimistic but will strive to be realistic and face the truth. Brain-injured patients do not recover fully from cognitive or personality dysfunction, but they do show improvement, and many show remarkable recovery. The role of treatment, in all its forms, is to facilitate and maximize that recovery process. In doing so, the patient moves from the relative status of personal dependence to independence, thereby becoming capable of making realistic commitments to work and family and once again reestablishing a sense of meaning in life.

In summary, psychotherapy after brain injury should attempt to:

1. Provide a model or models that help the patient understand what has happened to him or her
2. Help the patient deal with the meaning of the brain injury in his or her life
3. Help the patient achieve a sense of self-acceptance and forgiveness for himself or herself and others who have caused the accident
4. Help the patient make realistic commitments to work and interpersonal relations
5. Teach the patient how to behave in different social situations (to improve competence)
6. Provide specific behavioral strategies for compensating for neuropsychological deficits
7. Foster a sense of realistic hope

Elements of Psychotherapeutic Intervention

While there is no perfect way to conduct any form of psychotherapy with brain-injured patients, it has been my experience that certain conditions are necessary, but not sufficient in themselves, if the therapy is to be effective:

The patient needs simple explanations.
The explanations and behavioral coping strategies provided for them must be repetitively gone over.
Group pressure and group dynamics are needed to influence behavior. Individual treatment, by itself, is frequently not enough.
Individual insight and behavioral strategies are both employed to enhance coping skills.
Family members need to understand what the patient has learned and to follow through on this new learning in the home environment.

Each therapist has his or her own methods of relating to patients. Moreover, therapists enjoy different theoretical ideas as to what the patient needs to do in order to obtain significant benefit from psychotherapy. I consider the following to be useful guidelines:

Do not make it too easy for the patient to begin psychotherapy or a rehabilitation program. This may seem strange in light of the cognitive confusion that many of these patients experience, but the psychotherapeutic process with brain-injured patients, as well as with non-brain-injured patients, can be a draining experience and difficult to pursue. The patient and the therapist must deal frankly with the fact that formal psychotherapy may not be appropriate for a given patient at a given time. This should be discussed in some detail before therapy is attempted. It is important to emphasize to the patient (and frequently to the family) that if you (the therapist) make a commitment to work on these problems, the patient should make the same commitment. Some statement about a time-limited form of commitment is necessary too. This puts the commitment in a more realistic perspective.

Decide what constellation of individual and group psychotherapy sessions will be necessary. How much repetition of ideas will be needed? How much group feedback is necessary? How much individual support does the patient need? Ideally, working with the patient daily in individual and group psychotherapy helps get around eventual problems of abstraction and poor memory.

Plan what topics you are going to introduce in a given therapy session. Allow patients to bring up what is bothering them, but do not get sidetracked from discussing important issues. Also, teach the patients important information about their brain injury (this includes reviewing CT scans and basic neuroanatomy and neuropathology associated with their injuries).

Separate cognitive problems from emotional and motivational problems in therapy sessions, at least in the beginning. If possible, have designated cognitive therapy versus psychotherapy hours. The patient needs to reduce confusion about what is wrong and how to deal with it. The first group activity deals with cognitive functioning; the second must deal with personality disturbances.

In the group setting, provide a model of personality difficulties and teach patients how to cope with them. For example, we have emphasized the reactionary, neuropsychological, and characterological difficulties the patient experiences (see Chapter 3). This provides a simple explanation that can be understood and worked with. In addition, specific behavioral strategies for dealing with specific personality problems should be attempted if possible.

Reinforce awareness of deficits in self and others. This is crucial for eventual acceptance and motivation to compensate for residual difficulties.

Help each patient recognize how his or her personal background contributes to the rehabilitation progress. Patients may vary in their ability to use this kind of information. To the degree that the brain injury is put into perspective and they understand how they are coping with it, the better they are able to adjust and make a therapeutic alliance.

Point out the power of the group to reduce a sense of personal discomfort and to enhance a sense of belonging. Some patients will argue that they do not fit in with the other brain-injured patients. This is usually a defense against facing their own brain injury. Also, as patients begin to socialize with one another, it can be a sign that they are accepting their status as brain-injured people. If the group of patients avoid each other socially, this may reflect their avoidance of what has actually happened to them.

Obtain permission to give honest feedback (both painful and pleasant) within the context of the group setting. This is vital for honest work in a treatment environment.

Filter information and feedback to the patient in doses the patient can handle so that he or she can begin modifying socially incompetent behavior. Here behavioral modification techniques are invaluable.

Do not be afraid of using humor or analogies to get your point across, but do not lessen the seriousness of the business at hand. Your humanness and professionalism should come through. The patient should see you as a caring human being, but someone with specific knowledge and responsibilities to him or her and to others. I have been especially impressed with the power of analogies. Many brain-injured patients can instantly grasp something if the right analogy is given. We have found in group psychotherapy that the analogy of gestation and going through a pregnancy is quite useful in helping patients see where they are in the psychotherapeutic process. Many patients instantly know what is meant if they are told they are at five months in the process versus nine months. Similar analogies have been developed to help patients individually in the psychotherapy hour. Analogies get to the core issue with few words and powerful imagery. This approach is needed frequently with patients who have information-processing deficits, and it can be helpful even for those so-called normals who do not have such difficulties.

Be clear about the problems that need to be worked on, and periodically publicly review progress in writing.

Constantly remind yourself and the patient (1) that you will strive to be honest and face the truth about his or her strengths and weaknesses; (2) that you do not have all the answers but are committed to helping the patient change where possible; and (3) that there are no miracles in rehabilitation or psychotherapy — only hard work. If you and the patient are lucky, the intense effort will result in a substantial change in his or her adjustment.

Remind the patient that the pot of gold at the end of the rainbow is not necessarily happiness. The goal is to be independent, to be able to take care of one's needs and to be productive. As one mentally retarded patient stated, "I can work. I have freedom." If the patient is able to work, he or she will then have freedom, and with that comes the opportunity for enhanced interpersonal relationships. The secondary goal of love or interpersonal contact can be obtained, but there is no guarantee that this will take place.

A Schema for Conducting Psychotherapy after Brain Injury

Chapter 3 suggested that it is clinically useful to consider the personality disorders and resultant psychosocial difficulties of brain-injured patients along three dimensions: some disturbances are reactionary, some are neuropsychologically based, others are long-term and characterological in nature.

In conducting psychotherapy with brain-injured patients, individual and group psychotherapy is often necessary for them to deal realistically with their reactionary problems. Also in the context of individual and group psychotherapy, some of the long-term characterological problems might be dealt with, but this set of difficulties is notoriously difficult to treat using these methods, even in non-brain-injured patients.

Personality disorders that flow from disturbances in the neurology of thinking, memory, and perception are perhaps best dealt with by various forms of individual and group cognitively oriented exercises or retraining. The remainder of this chapter will discuss individual and group psychotherapy after brain injury as it relates to the reactionary and characterological problems. The importance of symbolism in psychotherapy will also be considered. A description of a cognitive group form of therapy aimed at dealing with the problem of socially inappropriate comments and tangentiality of language will be presented in Chapter 6. Chapter 6 will also describe examples of individual cognitive retraining, some of which deal with neuropsychologically mediated personality deficits.

Individual Psychotherapy

The public and some inexperienced psychotherapists often believe that individual psychotherapy is an expensive form of hand-holding in which one just tries to cheer up the patient (see Fig. 5.1). This is not what individual psychotherapy after brain injury is all about. Within the confines of a private, interpersonal exchange, the patient and therapist attempt to face the truth. What has gone wrong? What are the problems the patient experiences, and what are the likely causes? What steps might (and in some instances, should) be taken to cope with these problems and reestablish a sense of personal integrity and meaning in life?

By its nature, individual psychotherapy after brain injury will at times be a painful process. It is the responsibility of the therapist to stand toe-to-toe with the patient over the good times and the bad times. Much like a

Psychotherapy 75

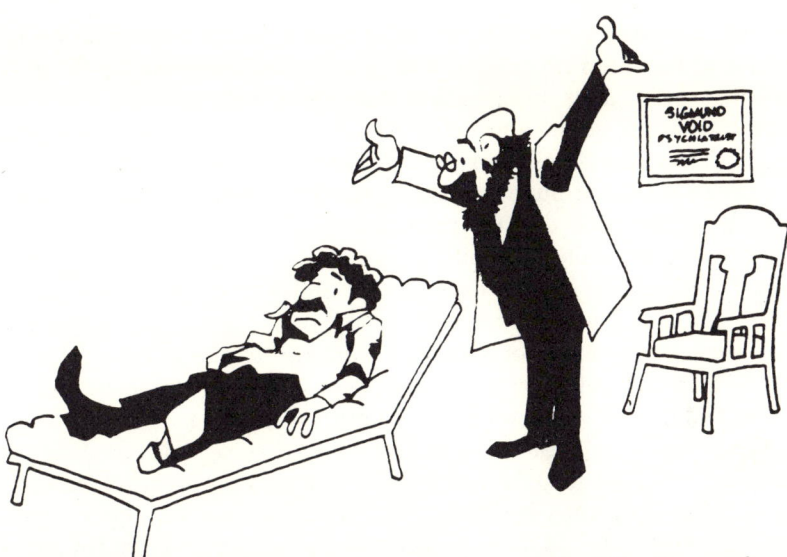

"What's the use of worrying? It never was worthwhile. So, pack up your troubles in your old kit bag and smile, smile, smile!"

Figure 5.1. Common Misperceptions of What Occurs in Psychotherapy. Reprinted by permission of the artist, Bill Hoest.

responsible parent, the therapist helps the patient understand the demands of life and learn how to meet those life challenges that are difficult to handle on his or her own. Because patients vary so much in terms of their reactionary, neuropsychologically based, and characterological personality difficulties, each patient needs some form of individual psychotherapy. There are patients who require minimal therapeutic intervention, but others may require years of psychotherapeutic work. Also, the models of behavior or explanations given to patients to help them cope with their difficulties vary because of these factors. To highlight this, two case examples will be presented in detail.

The first patient is a twenty-seven-year-old single white male who was a successful businessman prior to suffering a severe cranial trauma as a result of a small-plane crash. The patient had persistent headaches and ascribed all his behavioral problems to his headache pain several years postinjury. As he stated it, "My headaches caused me to fail." In the context of psychotherapy, the patient was able progressively to see that the opposite was true, that his failures in coping were apt to produce headaches. He was given a behavioral model for understanding how stress secondary to failure increases muscle tension and thereby produces headache pain, and he was asked to take specific behavioral steps to avoid experiencing failure and to keep his tension level within reasonable limits. When he followed this simple behavioral model, his headache pain decreased substantially and he was able to see that for years he had been avoiding the reality that he was not as good as he used to be. This was extremely painful for him to recognize, but eventually he could accept that his failures in life were caused by brain damage and not by the headaches.

Many traumatically head-injured patients, especially those who have been significantly impaired, explain their problems by pointing to things other than their brain damage, even several years posttrauma. All patients seek some explanation for what has happened to them. Psychotherapy should help such patients look honestly at how their abilities have been affected and how this may result in a number of problems.

The psychotherapy of the twenty-seven-year-old patient just described was relatively slow and was incorporated into the Neuropsychological Rehabilitation Program (see Chapter 6). As is the case with many brain-injured patients, he had to be worked with individually in order for him to focus his attention on some basic explanatory facts. By repetitively going over these facts, he began to incorporate the information. Then he could begin to discuss this insight during other rehabilitative activities, particularly those involving group interaction. It is important to emphasize that these insights must be understood by those who live with the patient and reinforced once the patient has completed rehabilitation. Memory difficulties make it necessary to rehearse frequently what has been previously learned and to have important others reinforce these insights. This helps the individual find more reasonable ways of coping with life and thereby reduce the catastrophic reaction.

The second example is a female physician who had suffered a hemorrhage of an arteriovenous malformation in the right parietal lobe. She had been a resident in radiology prior to her neurological insult. Because she had an excellent neurological recovery, she was allowed to go back to her residency several months after her neurological care, but to her surprise she discovered that she could not read x-rays as well as she used to. No one had prepared her for this predictable neuropsychological disturbance. She became progressively more upset with her failures in functioning and eventually dropped out of her residency program, taking instead a position in a small hospital as a statistician. Her neurologist eventually referred her for a neuropsychological evaluation because she felt the "patient was depressed." The neuropsychological workup revealed that this woman had many good residual neuropsychological skills. However, this woman now felt totally incompetent and was ashamed of her difficulties; she even avoided signing her name with the initials "M.D." after it.

In this case too it was necessary to begin psychotherapy on an individual basis. Because she felt so ashamed of her problems, it required a one-to-one interaction for her to begin to talk about her personal experiences after her surgery and understand what she was reacting to. Initially, the therapy consisted of describing her neuropsychological strengths and weaknesses. She was able to see that she did in fact have some abilities that were not being utilized. However, this stimulated a certain amount of psychological resistance. She had always seen herself as an extremely intelligent person, so when any part of her intelligence was affected, she saw her total value as an individual greatly diminished. Within the context of individual therapy, this erroneous belief was gently challenged. Because the therapist was able to show honest concern for this person and demonstrate that she still had much to offer, there was a surge of sexual feelings and sexual needs directed toward the therapist. Transference issues were dealt with. Within this context, the patient began discussing dream material that emphasized her feeling that something inside her had died. The dreams also revealed her shame and her sexual desires. Much of the work with this patient consisted of dream interpretation as it related to what she was now going through in coping with her residual neuropsychological problems. In many ways, the patient was treated with a psychoanalytically oriented approach, and this proved to be very helpful even though she had some brain dysfunction.

The point is that it does not matter what model is used to help a patient understand his or her difficulties in coping with a brain injury, provided the model makes sense to the therapist and the patient, given the circumstances of their lives and treatment. The key elements are that many brain-injured patients first need some individual contact in a private and protected manner to understand their difficulties, that they need explanations, and that they need to have those explanations gone over again and again. The competence of the therapist to go from one model to the next and gently help patients understand how their problems in coping with the effects of a brain injury are greatly compromising their life is of major importance. Once this individual work has begun, patients are in a much better position to deal with their reactionary problems and, in some instances, their long-term characterological problems in the context of a group setting. This is vital because unless patients are able to deal with the effects of their brain injury in interpersonal interactions, the degree of rehabilitation success is always limited.

Group Psychotherapy

Group psychotherapy with brain-injured patients is a fascinating and at times unpredictable phenomenon. Typically, two psychotherapists with training in clinical psychology and neuropsychology serve as the therapists. Anywhere from five to seven brain-dysfunctional patients constitute the group. It is usually better to have a closed group in which patients begin and end at the same time, because the patients need the security of a stable group interaction in order to deal with their personal tragedies in the most supportive manner.

One variable that makes group psychotherapy at times an unpredictable process is that one can never really tell what one patient is about to say to another. Sometimes what patients say to each other is quite helpful, but at other times the comments are off-target, inane, and even downright destructive. It is the responsibility of the psychotherapist to stay on top of what is being said and to cushion comments or modify them in order to help individual patients clarify their understanding of what is being said.

In the context of group psychotherapy with brain-injured patients, it is inevitable that the level of cognitive sophistication of patients will be quite variable. It is unlikely that there will be a homogeneous group of brain-dysfunctional patients. In fact, it is probably advantageous to have heterogeneity. This allows the individual patients to get a more realistic view of what their relative strengths and weaknesses are, compared with other individuals who have suffered brain injury. However, if one patient is at a very high level and another is at a very low level, some conflict is inevitable.

One purpose of group psychotherapy is to have patients understand how their brain injury influences their interpersonal interaction and to help them manage and cope with conflict within group settings. Their ability to do this is often a predictor of what they will be able to do once they leave rehabilitation. While group psychotherapy may seem unimportant to some patients, it has been my impression that once the group process begins these patients recognize, as do non-brain-injured patients, that the group experience is extremely influential. Patients frequently learn as much from each other as they do from what the therapists say. As a consequence, the group psychotherapeutic process is important.

In selecting members for group psychotherapy after brain injury, I found it useful to have them no younger than about eighteen years old and able at least to understand the communications of others. A few aphasic patients have been involved in group psychotherapy, but their receptive language skills have been good. Having more than one dysphasic patient in a group of this type, however, would be difficult and ill-advised. In addition, patients should have some minimal verbal skills; a Verbal IQ below 75 or 80 would rule someone out of this type of treatment. Finally, patients who are frankly psychotic or physically dangerous should not be in such groups. What is said can frequently be explosive, and if these patients have very little control of themselves they can act in ways that would destroy group cohesiveness.

The initial aim of group psychotherapy is to help the patients break down their sense of social isolation and to help them identify their present emotional and motivational difficulties. Perhaps the single long-term effect of brain injury is social isolation, and this is pointed out to the patients within the group process. It is also pointed out that patients frequently have a difficult time identifying their emotional and motivational disturbances, while those who live with them are highly sensitive to these problems. Frequently patients are asked to review lists of potential affective disturbances and identify those that might be most descriptive of themselves. This kind of structure often helps, particularly when the patients themselves cannot initiate a discussion of these problems or are greatly unaware of their difficulties.

Next, patients are helped to see the great similarity in their personality disorders even though differences do exist. They are helped to see that their brain injuries affect them all in predictable ways. Within this context, they are taught to see that how the brain injury affects their ability to interact with people greatly influences how people in turn react to them. Feelings are seen as important determinants of actions, and perhaps an intermediate goal or aim of group psychotherapy is for patients to begin to recognize this.

A long-term aim of group psychotherapy is for the patients to be able to identify their own form of the catastrophic reaction within a group setting and to discuss in a collective way how they may learn to cope with this difficulty. Several examples of the catastrophic reactions of preceding patients that had been in similar groups are given. As the catastrophic reaction is observed in patients within the context of group therapy or in other rehabilitative activities, it becomes a topic for open discussion. Some patients are also able to discuss their long-term personality characteristics in a group setting and how those characteristics influence the rehabilitation process. This becomes an extremely important example for others who have had difficulty discussing openly how brain injury has affected their emotional and motivational life. The ultimate aim of group psychotherapy is for patients to recognize and treat their emotional and motivational problems the same way they recognize and treat any other problems they experience following brain injury. In this way, it is hoped, the shame and embarrassment over these affective disturbances is reduced.

While there is no perfect way to conduct group psychotherapy, the following has proven to be helpful. Group psychotherapy typically begins by asking the patients to identify the name of the hour and its purpose. The scenario goes something like this: The name of the hour is group psychotherapy. The purpose of the hour is to talk about feelings, emotions, and motivations. We talk about feelings because how we feel determines in part how we act, and because that in turn determines how people react to us.

From here patients are asked to review the typical roadblocks to doing psychotherapy with brain-injured patients. In some instances I will state unabashedly that my colleagues tell me I may be wasting my time doing group psychotherapy with brain-injured patients because of these difficulties. The difficulties, which are stated and reviewed daily, are (1) that after brain injury patients have problems sustaining attention and therefore may miss what is being said; (2) that they have problems remembering what is said and therefore cannot integrate information from one session to the next; (3) that they have problems understanding what is being said and consequently may not grasp the point, so learning will go more slowly; and (4) many of them have trouble controlling their affective responses when confronted with negative information, and this can be disruptive to everyone. Once these problems are identified and recognized, they are fair game to discuss as they emerge within the context of group work. This allows patients to view these variables as important problems to cope with if group psychotherapy is going to be effective.

After the patients review this information, the psychotherapy hour begins. As indicated above, some agenda item, which the therapists take responsibility for introducing, is available for discussion, but patients are always given an opportunity to discuss what they consider relevant. Frequently, however, patients do not at first know what to bring up and will need guidance. Also, there is great variability in patients' ability to be introspective and to bring up useful information.

We have found it useful to prepare in advance a list of topics that could be discussed in group psychotherapy sessions for brain-injured patients. The exact order of topics is not always followed but it has proven to be a useful guideline.

Topic 1: Orientation to what group psychotherapy is all about and answering specific questions regarding why we attempt to do group psychotherapy. A handout is given to all patients and reviewed.

Topic 2: Patients are told that after brain injury people often have "emotional" reactions to what has happened to them as well as some basic change in their personality. Examples of this are given. Each patient is then asked: "What have been your emotional reactions to your brain injury?" Therapists look for the degree of insight and self-awareness and the capacity of the patient to deal with affective issues. A go-around technique is employed.

Topic 3: Patients are told that after brain injury people are often not fully aware of their emotional reactions and that relatives may see them differently from the way they see themselves. The question is then asked: "What do your relatives see as your emotional reaction to your brain injury?" Again, degree of insight, degree of empathy, and the degree to which the patient can deal with emotional issues is assessed.

Topic 4: A definition of personality (which includes basic interest, attitudes, values, and interpretation of life) is given in simple terms. Patients are then asked: "How has your personality changed since your brain injury?"

Topic 5: Again patients are reminded that relatives often see things differently from patients. The question is asked: "How do your relatives see your personality at the present time? Do they think there has been any change? What is their evidence for this?"

Topic 6: Patients often do not understand relatives' motivations or reactions to them. The question is raised: "If relatives could change anything in your emotional reaction or your personality following the injury, what would they change and why?" An effort is made to get patients to start thinking about their relatives' perspective as opposed to their own perspective.

Topic 7: The same question as that in Topic 6 is raised, but now it is phrased this way: "If you could change your emotional reaction or personality following your brain injury, what would you change and why?" The purpose is to see the degree to which patients are starting to become objective about what their problems are and what problems should be changed first.

Topic 8: The topic of a catastrophic reaction is now formally introduced. A description of the catastrophic reaction in various forms is presented. Patients are asked to describe their own form of the catastrophic reaction. Emphasis is placed on the natural basis of this reaction, and research and theoretical information concerning it is provided the patients.

Topic 9: Patients are then presented with empirical information regarding emotional and motivational problems that have been reported in the literature on head-injury patients. They are presented with lists of problems (particularly Roberts 1979) and asked to identify what problems in the list are true for them. This provides more structure than the open-ended interview questions that were asked earlier. (Note: At various times, pertinent articles or films [e.g., a *Wall Street Journal* article on head injury or on the return to work after severe head injury, or a film from the University of California at San Diego on computer graphics of the brain] are introduced and used to stimulate or supplement discussions.)

Topic 10: After the patient goes over each list, the go-around technique is again applied, and individuals are asked to comment on what the other patients may have left off on their own lists. This is the first time patients are asked to confront one another and give both positive and negative feedback as to the accuracy of a patient's description of his or her own emotional characteristics. Note that this occurs several weeks into the rehabilitation program, in order to minimize resistance to doing group psychotherapy with these individuals.

Topic 11: The point that brain injury can change parts of an individual's personality is presented. A review of functional neuroanatomy is given, and the patients' CT scans are reviewed. Their medical records are described in terms of what is known about the neuropsychology of emotional and motivational disturbances. This follows Topic 10, where patients are confronted with one another, and provides a cooling-off period.

Topic 12: Patients are now asked to talk about their emotional reaction in relation to their neuropsychological deficits: How do they feel about specific deficits they experience?

Topic 13: Patients are told about the importance of giving feedback to one another regarding their day-to-day functioning. While they have done this in other hours, such as in cognitive group therapy, now is the time to do this with regard to emotional functioning. Again, a go-around technique is used.

Topic 14: Patients again list emotional difficulties they have had following their brain injury. After reviewing this, patients give feedback to one another as to what each may have left off his or her list. This is another confrontation technique, but usually by this time there is greater rapport and therapeutic alliance.

Topic 15: The problem of body image after brain injury is focused on.

Topic 16: The topic of self-confidence after brain injury is focused on.

Topic 17: The topic of paranoid ideation is focused on.

Topic 18: The topic of denial of illness is focused on.

Topic 19: The topic of sexual dysfunction is addressed.

Topic 20: The topic of social isolation and withdrawal is addressed.

Topic 21: The problems in dealing with spouse and children are addressed.

Topic 22: The topic of dealing with relatives other than spouse and children is addressed.

Topic 23: Feelings concerning work and going back to work at a lower level are discussed.

Topic 24: Patients are asked if they could conduct group psychotherapy more like psychiatric patients as opposed to neurological patients. This is done to determine what they have learned from their group experience in handling their problems with less structure.

It is important to recognize that the group psychotherapeutic process with brain-injured patients follows many of the rules described by students of group psychotherapy with psychiatric patients (see Yalom 1970). Scapegoats frequently emerge within the context of the group process. Some patients are identified as the odd ones, the ones who do not fit or are troublemakers. Cliques may develop, as in the case of certain patients allying themselves with others. The dynamics of these interactions can give the rehabilitation therapists clues to the normal methods of adjusting that the various brain-dysfunctional patients utilize.

Within the context of group psychotherapy, it is also likely that some patients will be more able to articulate certain dynamic issues, which can be very helpful to other patients who are less able to put into words what they are experiencing. One example of this is a poem written by the woman physician who had suffered an arteriovenous malformation, described earlier in this chapter:

Group Psychotherapy

In group psychotherapy we sit
Wondering where in life we can fit,
Which of our feelings should we admit?
And which hold with bridle and bit?
Once some of us on the head were hit.
Sometimes we feel we were hit by shit.
Some of us had good jobs that we quit;
Are we able to do more than knit?
When we fail again, our teeth we grit,
Sometimes words are hard to spit,
Is there more to life than this big pit?

This poignant poem has been useful for many groups of brain-injured patients. It highlights some of the negative reactions that patients experience while doing group psychotherapy, and it also highlights their worries and thoughts, which are frequently difficult to bring out within the group context. This type of artistic expression is seen in many types of brain-injured patients despite the severity of their injuries. When it emerges within the group psychotherapy context, it can be a powerful ally in helping patients deal with the issues of meaning in their lives after brain injury. Symbolism and artistic expression can be important tools in the treatment of brain-injured patients.

The Importance of Symbolism in the Therapeutic Process

Since most brain-injured patients show some impairment of the abstract attitude (Goldstein 1942), the importance of using symbolism in psychotherapy is frequently overlooked. Symbols often convey a unique mixture of ideas and feelings that cannot be put into simple words or gestures.

Jungian therapists have long been aware of this (see Jung 1964), and some of them have applied this insight to psychotherapeutic work with severely ill patients, including brain-injured children (Bach 1969). While various art forms can be used to facilitate the psychotherapeutic process, drawings may be especially helpful to brain-injured patients who have a minimum of education or who have aphasic difficulties.

In a remarkable drawing (Fig. 5.2), one young man was able to convey his experience of what it was like to be brain damaged. The patient drew a lateral view of the brain with an electrical cord coming from its base. The cord is partially disconnected from the wall socket, from which fly sparks and smoke. The patient remarks that he feels as though the energy that is coming from the wall has been partially disconnected. He does not have the same vitality or the same clarity of thought he used to have. The smoke reflects his confusion, his inability to see clearly what is happening to him. His next drawing (Fig. 5.3) reflects the powerful connection between cognitive confusion and feeling states. Many of his humanoid figures, who have holes in their heads, are unable to establish a clear facial expression. When patients are greatly confused, they are not clear about what their feeling states are. This is extremely important to get across to patients who are severely impaired. When the confusion subsides, feelings of depression or deep sorrow often emerge (see Fig. 5.3, third figure from the right).

Such drawings can help patients convey ideas necessary for facing the existential realities of their life. As patients review their pictures, they gain an important insight into their lives, and this can help them modify their behavior and further reduce their cognitive confusion.

A second patient, with a persistent aphasia, drew himself at the end of his rehabilitation program (Fig. 5.4). He symbolizes his hemiplegia and cognitive confusion. Only at the end of his rehabilitation program was he able to draw this. Prior to that time, all he felt he needed was bigger and better speech and language therapy. At the end of the program, he sees a choice point in life and chooses to follow the path that leads to "God." No matter what one's religious persuasion, the concept of God has extraordinary psychological significance. God can represent a coming to grips with reality, a connecting of one's self to something beyond a limited biological existence. When this takes place, the patient has a sense of integration and individuation (in Jungian terms) that is necessary for acceptance of the tragedy in his or her life. The patient can then move ahead psychologically.

Two other drawings (Figs. 5.5 and 5.6) come from a thirteen-year-old boy who suffered a clearly documented left hemisphere injury. Prior to his injury, this child was exceedingly bright, and after the injury he maintained outstanding nonverbal problem-solving skills. For example, his WISC-R Block Design postinjury was a scale score of 17, despite a clear

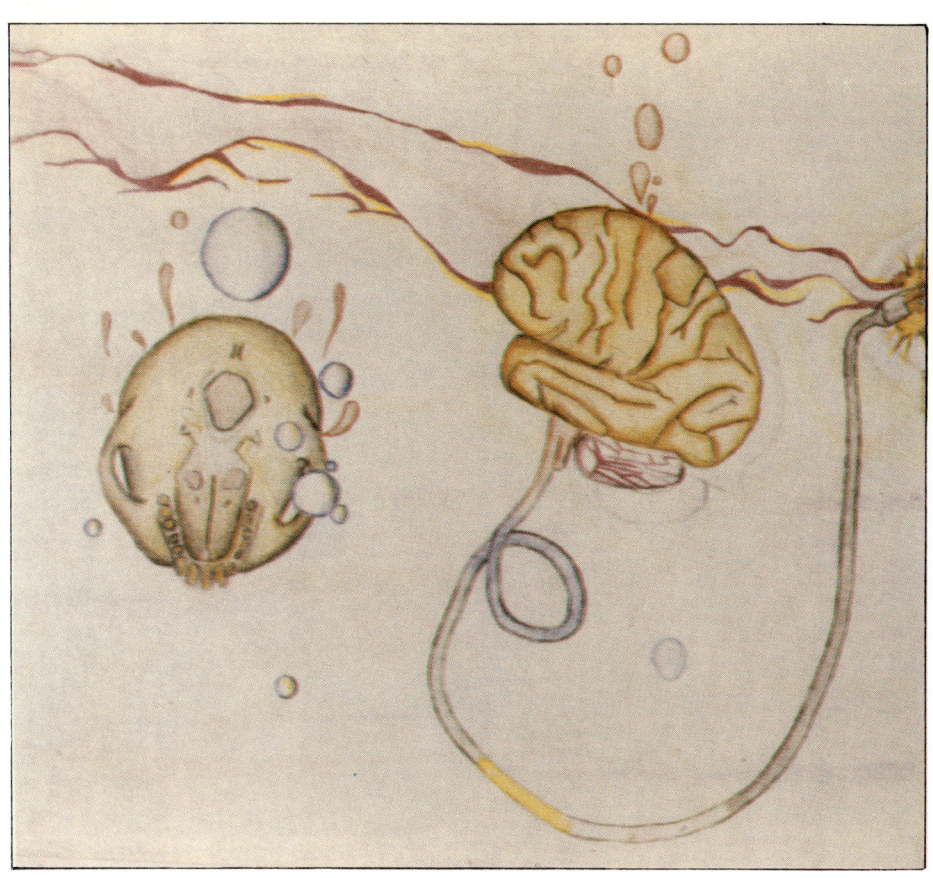

Figure 5.2. Spontaneous Drawing by a Young Adult Brain-injured Patient

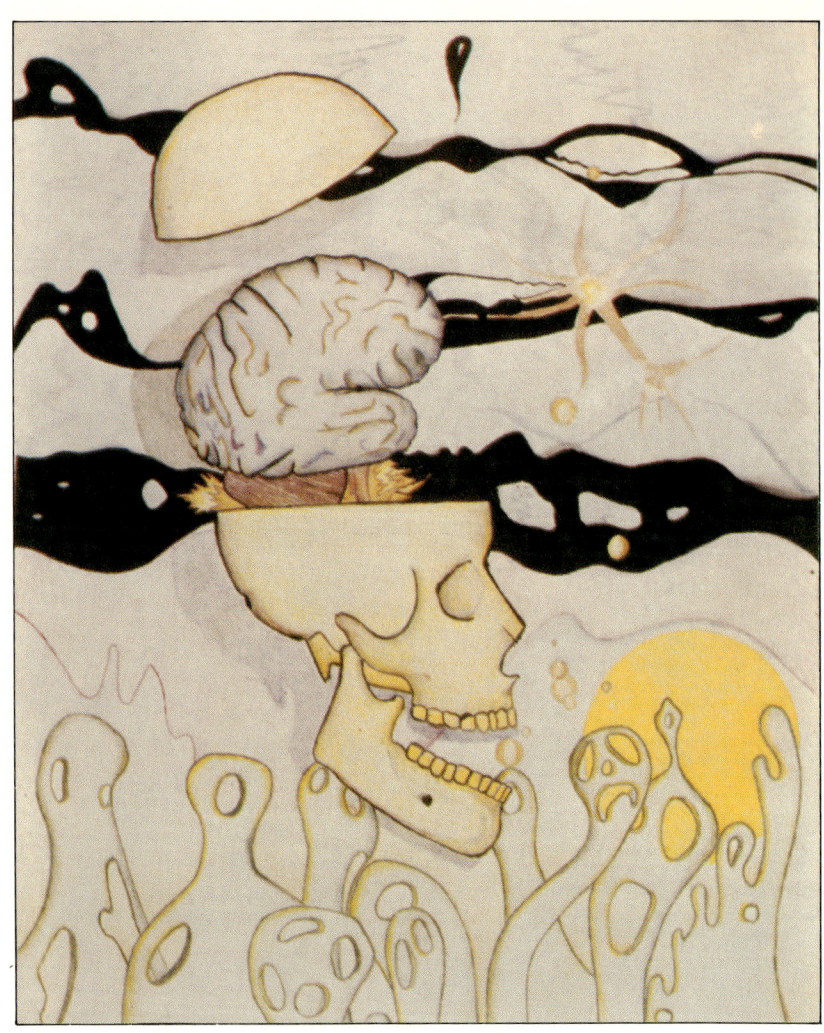
Figure 5.3. A Second Drawing from the Same Patient

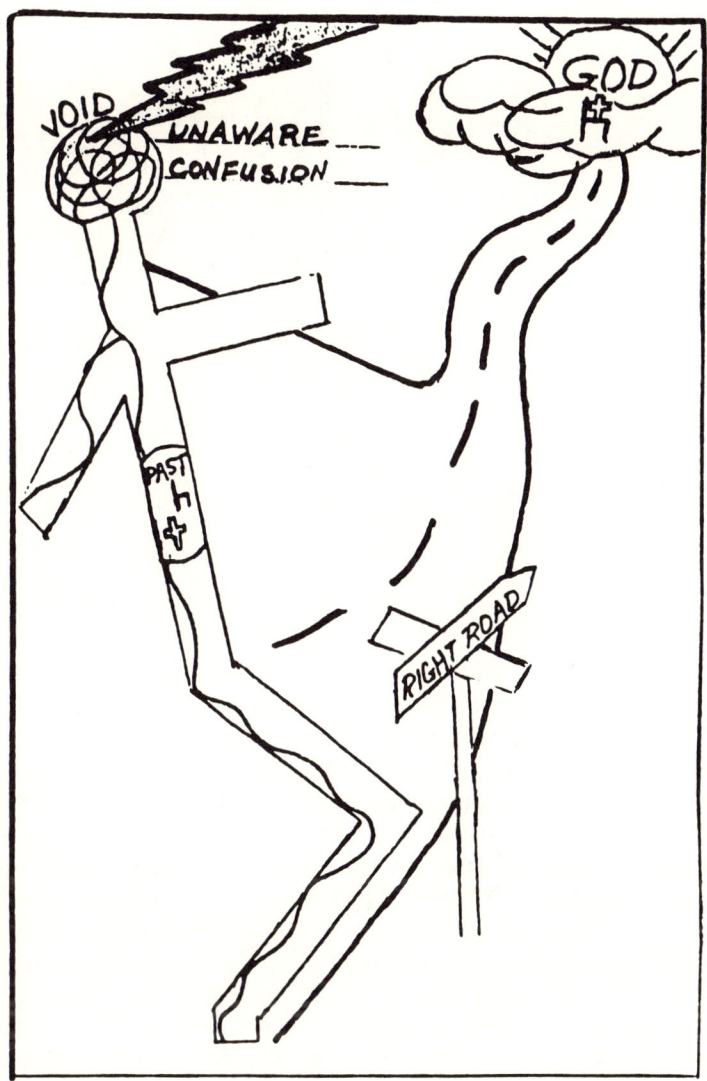

Figure 5.4. Spontaneous Drawing by a Traumatic Head-Injury Patient at the Completion of a Rehabilitation Program

fluent dysphasia. This boy was worked with primarily from a cognitive remediation point of view. One day, unsolicited, he presented the drawing shown in Figure 5.5, stating that his school assignment was to draw a picture using perspective. The picture has rich symbolism. First, it is entitled "In the Twilight Zone." Many brain-injured patients, despite their retained level of intelligence, recognize that their contact with reality has been

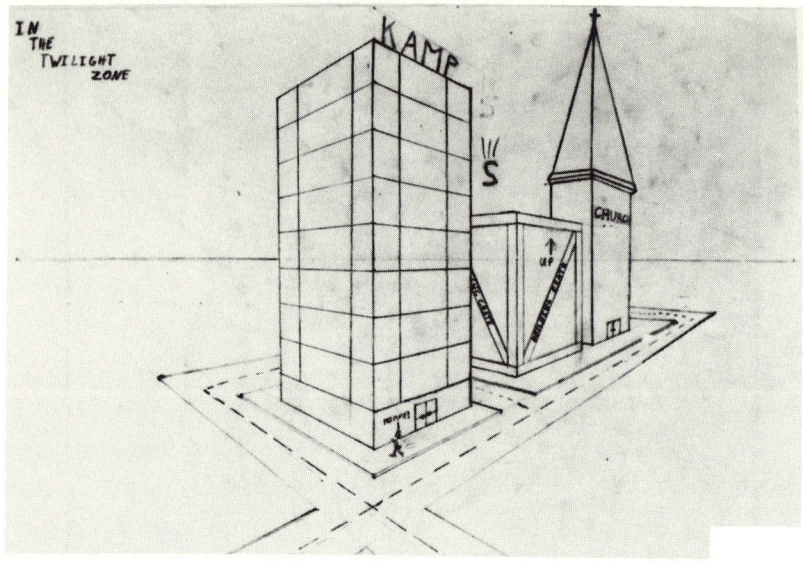

Figure 5.5. Drawing by an Adolescent Head-injured Boy

changed, and they are confused by it. Second, his family's last name is placed on top of a large building with the last letter falling from it. At first, this was interpreted as reflecting his feelings toward his language disorder (i.e., the difficulties in keeping letters together). Later, however, he made it clear that there was a much more personal meaning attached to this symbolism. He was angered and frustrated with the therapists' earlier interpretative comments, which were apparently seen as insensitive and intrusive. He stated to his mother that there were five letters in their last name and five members in his family. He was the youngest (i.e., the last) and the letter *S* represented him and his feeling that he was "falling away" from the rest of the family following his injury. Bach (1969) emphasized the importance of the number of things depicted in the drawings of children and that cursory interpretation should be avoided.

In the same picture this child also drew a building in a crate and a church next to it. The former conveys the feeling of a "twilight zone," the latter introduces the theme of God. Religious themes are frequently seen in many left-hemisphere-injury patients' drawings and art work. Finally, the picture shows a little boy calling for "Mommy." The need to be reconnected with a secure, loving environment is a common need of many brain-injured patients, despite their inability to state this verbally.

The themes depicted in this child's drawing were a part of his experience that was not verbally reported when interacting with therapists. He usually

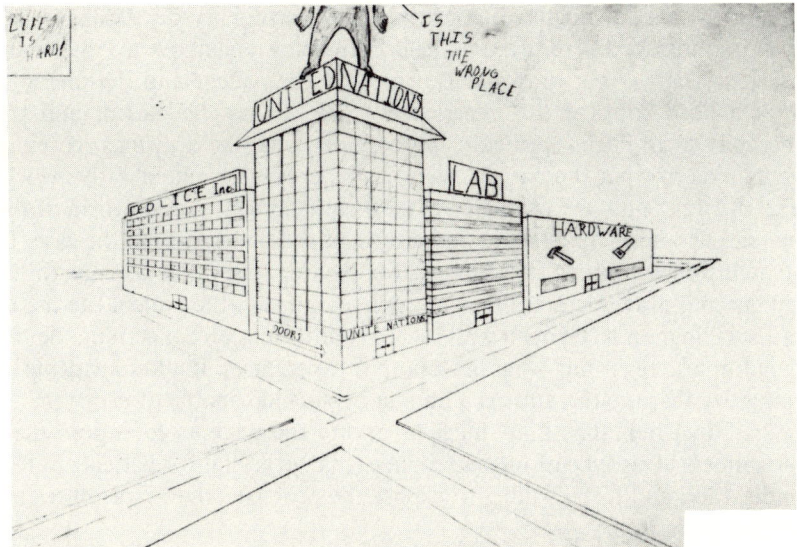

Figure 5.6. A Second Drawing from the Same Patient

appeared to be self-confident, independent, and optimistic, but his drawings showed that he was experiencing another realm not described in typical social interaction. Understanding this other realm allows the therapist to deal with the patient and the family in a more sensitive and therapeutic manner.

The second drawing by this youth, entitled "Life Is Hard" (Fig. 5.6), was obtained a few weeks later. The patient is aware of his struggle to improve his cognitive and language functioning and how difficult it can be. He draws a figure similar to King Kong without the head and neck. The figure is asking the question "Is this the wrong place?" The ape is standing on the United Nations building rather than on the expected Empire State building. At first, this comment was thought to reflect the boy's cognitive confusion, but because this was the last drawing spontaneously presented to his therapist, another interpretation is possible. Perhaps the boy was feeling that he was in the wrong place for his psychotherapy or cognitive remediation. The interpretation of the preceding drawing (Fig. 5.5) had clearly upset him, and the therapist subsequently did not see him in regular psychotherapy sessions because the boy did not want to be seen in psychotherapy after this. The second drawing may convey the boy's need for further discussion and for a therapist that can deal with the complex issues he experiences.

Symbolism can be important in work with brain-injured patients, whatever their level of cognitive confusion and personality disturbance. The drawings included here, from patients both below and above average in intelligence, show that drawings can provide the patient and the therapist with a hard copy of life experiences. This allows the patient and the therapist to go back repeatedly and consider what the drawings represent as a guide to what the patient needs in the course of rehabilitative work. The therapist must be willing to enter the phenomenological world of the patient, as well as understand the scientific facts that surround the case. In some instances, it may be necessary for the therapist to sit down with the patient and draw pictures. This not only conveys to the patient the therapist's willingness to be open with regard to information concerning the patient but also regarding what the therapist experiences. It allows patients to recognize that the therapist is a human being and capable of exposing his or her own humanness as much as asking the patients to expose their humanness. This type of interpersonal exchange is vital for patients to feel understood and to be willing to expose the problems they experience following brain injury.

Predictable Psychotherapeutic Problems

While it is impossible to discuss in great detail the various psychotherapeutic issues that have been addressed with brain-dysfunctional patients, some classical problems deserve comment. The purpose of this section is to alert clinicians to these issues as they unfold with various brain-dysfunctional patients and to point out areas that might be addressed within the therapeutic context. In addition, this section emphasizes that not all problems after brain injury can be successfully treated with psychotherapy. There is a mystique that psychotherapy can resolve all the reactionary or characterological problems of brain-dysfunctional patients, but this is not the case. However, if the therapist has some understanding of what problems are more amenable to change and what problems are not, then both the therapist and the patient can proceed with the psychotherapeutic venture with realistic expectations.

One classical problem that emerges concerns the adjustment of the brain-injured person after divorce. Because a brain-injured person is permanently changed and his or her level of competency and personality may be altered in a negative direction, many spouses eventually separate from the patient or significantly alter the interpersonal relationship. Many brain-injured patients can be helped to face divorce. An example is one man who had suffered a rupture of a right parietal aneurysm. He worked hard to get back to gainful employment, but once he had achieved this, his wife confronted him and asked for a divorce. He felt this was unfair and was very angry with her. He turned to drinking for several weeks, and psychotherapy consisted mainly of pouring him hot coffee. Over an extended period of time, however, he was able to face the reality of what had happened because his rehabilitation had helped him become truly independent. With that, he was able to improve his physical appearance greatly and maintain a job that would put him in contact with others. As of this writing, he has been dating and has established a stable interpersonal life. Follow-up with this patient suggested that he had adjusted to his brain injury and his divorce because he was able to move from a dependent state to an independent state.

The brain-injured patient who protests that psychotherapy is not helpful presents another problem. Many times, psychotherapy touches on painful issues that brain-injured patients, as well as non-brain-injured patients, do not want to face. At times, patients will protest that psychotherapy is useless and has no value. One patient, in the context of our neuropsychological rehabilitation program, announced one day that he had been coming to psychotherapy for several weeks and it was of no use to him. I responded by stating that perhaps psychotherapy should not be attempted with brain-injured patients because if I had been in a group psychotherapy program on a day-in and day-out basis for several weeks I certainly would have learned something about myself. I commented, tongue-in-cheek, that maybe psychotherapy has nothing to offer brain-injured people because they simply cannot learn from their mistakes. At this point, the patient protested that psychotherapy was extremely important and refused to allow it to be deleted from the program. Calling the patient's bluff on the effectiveness of psychotherapy is sometimes necessary. It allows the patient to realize that you are willing to listen to criticisms but will still try to maintain facing the truth with patients over the problems they experience.

Another frequently encountered problem is how to deal with the "nice guy" brain-injured patient who irritates both staff and family. Some brain-injured patients have premorbid personality characteristics that result in their being overly polite and overly solicitous to others. This can be irritating to staff, fellow patients, and the patient's family. It is painful to have to bring this to a patient's attention, but it is necessary to do so. Underneath the "nice guy" attitude is often a great deal of resentment or anger. One patient was helped to recognize that this super-syrupy approach to life was turning everybody off. With this, he took a much more realistic stance with his wife. They went through several ups and downs and were seriously contemplating divorce, but he was able to get back to gainful employment, work through this problem by looking at his underlying anger, and reconstitute his marriage.

The brain-injured patient who misperceives the environment is another classic problem. Patients who have frontal and/or temporal lobe injuries often do not get the point of what is being said. They can greatly misinterpret the intentions or actions of others, particularly puns or jokes, taking what people are saying literally and becoming angry with them. Helping these patients recognize that they are thinking too concretely and that they must broaden their scope in order to not misjudge others is important. When this type of misperception comes from impairment of the abstract attitude, much can be done to help improve a patient's perception of the environment. When the misperception has a paranoid flavor, it may mean that there is a temporal lobe disorder with associated amnestic difficulties, which is much more difficult to treat and in our experience has never been adequately dealt with.

A fifth problem has to do with helping the brain-injured patient face cognitive deficits. Perhaps the ultimate goal of all rehabilitation after brain injury is to face life as it really is rather than how one wishes it would be. One patient who initially came to us felt that all he really needed was more effective speech and language therapy. Progressively, however, he came to realize that he had many more problems than his aphasic disorder (this patient was the one who drew Fig. 5.4). By the time he finished rehabilitation, he was able to accept the very severe cognitive deficits he had and still found meaning in life without giving up or becoming hostile toward others.

Working through the psychological resistance to treatment and dealing with the problem of transference comprise another problem clinicians may have to deal with. Goldstein (1942) recognized that brain-injured patients, like psychotic patients, tend to make intense and immediate transference, which can be both positive and negative. It is common for brain-injured patients to think that their therapists are "the best." Therapists who easily accept this form of distortion can look forward to experiencing a strong dose of negative transference later in treatment. Related to this, some patients can have intense sexual feelings toward therapists. Therapists must recognize this when it emerges and deal with it appropriately, helping the patient recognize that sexual feelings may reflect something more basic. These patients frequently feel that when someone understands them or cares for them, it is only natural that they would show physical affection toward the therapist as well. Being able to deal with this problem at various levels of cognitive retraining and psychotherapy is important. It allows the patient to sustain the drive and motivation to be with the therapist, but the therapist should utilize this motivation to keep the patient on track about what the relationship actually is, instead of maintaining unrealistic ideas about some total engulfing relationship.

Anxiety and depressive reactions of various brain-injured patients are another common problem area. Anxiety is often stimulated when the patient cannot cope in an environment. By helping patients understand what environments they can cope with, one can greatly decrease anxiety. Also, depressive reactions can be dealt with when patients recognize that they have retained strengths as well as weaknesses. Many patients who are unable to cope with their depressive reactions experienced significant problems with depression prior to the injury.

Another problem that may have to be dealt with is difficulty in getting patients to forgive themselves. Some patients, no matter how hard one works with them, cannot forgive themselves or others for what has happened. When there is both a severe amnestic disorder and paranoid ideation, the combination can produce an angry patient unwilling to change his or her perspective. With such individuals there is often a strong underlying premorbid problem that is unleashed by the brain injury. If the brain injury takes away the patient's ability to cope with the problems experienced in life prior to the injury, the patient has no way of feeling good about himself or herself or supplementing painful perceptions of self. These individuals often require long-term care and frequently alienate family members.

Still another problem is presented when a paranoid patient becomes violent. Rapidly confronting a paranoid patient may indeed stimulate violence, and this can become a major burden for family and therapists. Paranoid patients can be physically dangerous. They often require a protected environment with minimal confrontation. One such patient we treated early in our program became much worse in his day-to-day functioning when confronted on a constant basis. It has been our experience that this type of patient frequently does not benefit from the type of rehabilitation described in this volume. Other methodologies need to be developed to handle such individuals in the future.

Failure to overcome the "take care of me" attitude is another classic problem that is likely to come up. While many brain-injured patients feel helpless, it has been found that some manifested a "take care of me" attitude prior to their brain injury. One patient, who was adopted early in life, felt strongly that the therapists should take care of him. He was childlike and demanding, but when this was pointed out to him, it only met with more resistance—presumably due to premorbid personality structure prior to the brain injury. We were never able to overcome this problem when it appeared in intense forms.

One more problem is failure to overcome the self-destructive component of the patient—the problem of suicide. Since the beginning of our intensive neuropsychological rehabilitation at Presbyterian Hospital, only one patient eventually took his life, a patient who had suffered carbon monoxide poisoning. Initial diagnostic inquiries as to whether the patient's accident was a suicide attempt were hotly denied by everyone, including the patient and family. After about six to nine months of work with this patient, however, it finally emerged that the "accident" was indeed a suicide attempt. The patient did relatively well from a cognitive retraining point of view, but as he improved in his cognitive functioning he started to become more depressed, resulting in inpatient hospitalization. At that time we did not know whether electroconvulsive therapy (ECT) would be helpful, but it was attempted. The effect of ECT was to undo the effects of cognitive retraining. Within a short period of time, the patient was again in a confused state, but no longer depressed. Eventually the confusion lifted and the patient became depressed once again. After being discharged and going to another state where he was reportedly to live with a relative, he eventually took his life. Suicide is certainly a major problem for brain-injured patients, but it may be more related to premorbid personality problems than to the brain injury per se.

The final classical type of problem has to do with the self-destructive patient who does not reach suicide but continues to alienate others. A large number of head-injury patients fit in this category. They are not so self-destructive that they ultimately take their lives, but their premorbid characteristics suggest significant interpersonal difficulties. They often enjoy upsetting others, and bringing this out in the context of group and individual psychotherapy produces a considerable emotional effect, frequently tears and sadness. Yet they are tied to this basic view of themselves and way of interacting with others. One such patient worked with us for an entire year. While we understood these dynamics, he was unable to change them. He remained unemployed after intensive effort to get him a job.

As is evident from the above, many of the failures in psychotherapy with brain-injured patients are seen in individuals who had major psychiatric problems before their injury, but not all these patients showed obvious signs of such problems before the injury. Their jobs and cognitive skills allowed them to keep those problems under control, but when the brain injury undercut their cognitive abilities, the underlying psychiatric disturbances emerged. In contrast, the patients who seem to benefit most from psychotherapy are those who are committed to becoming independent, can take a realistic view of themselves, can see their strengths and weaknesses, and can work at cognitive remediation.

Education, Social Support, and Psychotherapy of Family Members

Because brain-injured patients often are not fully aware of their residual neuropsychological and personality disturbances, family members may initiate professional consultation and intervention. The emphasis is always on getting the patient the help he or she needs, yet once the patient does receive rehabilitative help, family members frequently also require consultation. Many family members reject this either because of financial considerations or because they feel they must be strong for the patient. But once family members are given an opportunity to be educated concerning the nature of the problems their relative has and the methods of intervention, a broad array of topics is opened up. In addition to knowing "what's wrong" with the patient, the family members need to know what steps to take to manage the patient at home. Sometimes this results in simple, practical activities. In other instances it is very difficult to teach families to do this because there may be a high degree of psychopathology within the family structure itself. Also, some families simply lack the education or the sophistication to apply certain kinds of behavioral approaches in managing a difficult patient.

Nevertheless, relatives need to be educated, and this is usually accomplished in two or three ways. First, the neuropsychological test findings should be shared with them. Second, if the patient is involved in a rehabilitation program, the family should be given a thorough orientation to that program. A full-day orientation program helps family members go through exactly what patients go through. This is extremely helpful to understanding the nature of the treatments. Finally, family members need to have an opportunity to talk with members of other patients' families so that they can learn how others cope with brain-injured people.

Developing a social support system is a second, very important activity with family members. Bond (1983) summarized research findings regarding the impact of head injury on family systems. He noted that it is primarily the mental (including personality) disturbances that are most distressful to family members. Moreover, he cited studies that indicate that with the passage of time there is frequently an increase in personality disturbances with brain-injured patients. In our own research, we observed this to be true (Fordyce et al. 1983). As time goes on, therefore, family members need more help in understanding what is wrong with the patient and how to cope with it. Social support systems allow individuals to begin to talk about their personal reactions to a brain-injured patient. Family members often resist doing this, again feeling that they should be strong for the patient. They typically experience hostility, guilt, depression, and despair, as documented by Bond (1983) and others.

Hostility comes from the fact that the patients are very demanding and frequently interfere with other family members' getting their needs met. Because the person is handicapped or impaired, there is an assumption that all family members should bend to meet the needs of the patient. This can be done for a period of time, but since the problems of head injury are long-term, this eventually takes its toll. Family members sooner or later become angry or downright hostile toward the brain-injured patient. They often feel that the patient could do better if he or she only tried harder. When they realize that the problems go beyond just motivation, they are apt to feel guilty about their reactions to brain-injured relatives. Depression and despair typically follow guilt.

It has been our experience that family members need to understand their personal reactions to a brain-injured patient and take practical steps to avoid the ultimate depression and despair. For example, one child of a head-injury patient recently sought psychotherapy, saying that she was distressed because she did not feel the love toward her mother that she believed she should. Her mother had been injured when this young woman was thirteen years old. Throughout her adolescence, she did not get the support or help that she would have liked from her mother over the typical issues of dating, career choices, and so on, so she began to withdraw from her mother and relied on others for that type of support. The family was very religious and could not tolerate the feeling that everybody was not closely affiliated with everyone else. This produced notable guilt in the young woman, and she was unable to talk with other family members regarding it.

Something similar can also happen to spouses. People are apt to be afraid to talk about their lack of love for a spouse because they are concerned that once they discuss this in private it will lead automatically to divorce or separation. Yet in some instances spouses and children need to have individual psychotherapy to work through their relationship with a brain-injured patient. They need help in clarifying what they can expect from the patient and what needs they will have to meet outside the relationship. This is not much different from facing any tragedy of life and going through the mourning process.

While we are beginning to understand the problems that head-injury patients cause for family members, we have not fully explored the types of psychotherapy that would be most helpful in dealing with these patients and family members. The literature on psychotherapy with relatives who are going through other chronic illnesses should be explored in this regard.

The Reactions of Professional Staff to Brain-injured Patients

Working with brain-injured patients can be fatiguing and frustrating. The patients' cognitive confusion, inappropriate comments, difficulties in new learning, and emotional lability make it difficult for staff who have made a commitment to work with them. In fact, the professional staff experience everything the families go through in living with brain-injured patients if they make a true commitment to the patients.

The staff must therefore enter into a fair and honest relationship with the patients if they are not going to be burned out by their rehabilitative work. Usually having staff make a time-limited commitment helps. Staff can understand what their responsibilities are for a given time and are expected to make an intense commitment during this interval. However, they should not be expected to keep working with patients indefinitely. For many staff, this is just too demanding.

Second, the staff need a social support system that allows them some break from their intensive interaction with patients. (This is true for the family as well.) This break can take many forms. The staff may be involved in administrative or research work during the day or at the end of the week. It may also take the form of rotating out of rehabilitative work into other types of patient care for periods of time. This allows the staff to feel some relief of the burden involved in working with these patients.

In addition, the staff need to have experiences that allow them to grow professionally. Their ability to learn something new from the patients they treat is vital to keeping the staff energetic. Helping them conduct clinical research on the patients they treat can be helpful in this regard.

Finally, helping the staff understand their personal reactions to patients and why they chose rehabilitative work in the first place is crucial. Rehabilitation therapists have a need to help and care for others. If patients do not respond to the staff's conscious or unconscious expectations, the staff can become bitter, angry, solicitous, and so on. Periodic staff consultation with a consulting psychiatrist has proven helpful in clarifying patients' needs versus staff needs. If the staff can get their needs met in a way that does not exploit patients, the rehabilitative process can continue in a realistic and motivated manner. One cannot expect patients to maintain these characteristics (motivation and realism) unless the rehabilitation staff also embrace the same experiences. To achieve this, one must select staff carefully and have a work setting that encourages these values.

Summary

Psychotherapy after brain injury can be vital if reasonable adaptation to a severe illness is to be accomplished. Certainly the patient needs help dealing with personality and cognitive disturbances after brain injury. In addition, the family members and the hospital staff must come to grips with their affective difficulties in living or working with these patients. If the patient, the family, and therapists can have their needs met and ultimately behave in their best interests, a truly curative process takes place. If there is interpersonal exploitation at any level of the interaction, the therapeutic relationship is corroded and the patient has major difficulties facing reality.

While the outcome of psychotherapy is certainly variable, as described by the examples of successes and failures, the goal is to help the patient make a greater commitment to life. Family and staff also can be helped to make realistic commitments to the patient. If this is done, substantial improvement in the patient's quality of life after significant brain injury occurs and brings maximum functional recovery.

CHAPTER 6
The Neuropsychological Rehabilitation Program at Presbyterian Hospital, Oklahoma City

George P. Prigatano and David J. Fordyce

The preceding chapters described the long-range cognitive and personality problems of young adult brain-injured patients. They also broadly discussed the concepts of cognitive retraining and psychotherapy after brain injury. The present chapter describes in some detail the rehabilitation environment and program from which those ideas emerged.

The Neuropsychological Rehabilitation Program (NRP) at Presbyterian Hospital in Oklahoma City began in response to the needs of young adult brain-injured patients who were essentially independent in their daily functioning but were unable to return to a productive life-style. These patients have cognitive and personality disturbances even though their physical and gross neurological recovery was good. As a group, these patients can easily become confused and experience residual memory deficits with associated problems in learning new information (Chapter 1); they are tangential in their thoughts and comments (Chapter 2); and they are generally impulsive and at times irritable (Chapter 3). Eventual social withdrawal and isolation from others was a common occurrence. The ultimate impact of this was that the patient typically became unemployed, progressively lost pretrauma friendships and relationships, and became a significant burden to himself or herself as well as to the family and society (Oddy et al. 1978; Weddell et al. 1980).

There has been a growing recognition that these cognitive and personality disturbances after severe head injury are not adequately dealt with by traditional rehabilitation methods (Bond 1975; Bond and Brooks 1976; Fahy et al. 1967; Bruckner and Randle 1972; Walker 1972; Najenson et al. 1974). The NRP was developed to help patients return to a higher level

---
An earlier version of this chapter will appear in B. Caplan and G. Bray, eds., *Handbook of Contemporary Rehabilitation Psychology* (Springfield, Ill.: Charles C Thomas, in press). Reprinted by permission of the publisher.

of psychosocial functioning given the principles outlined for cognitive retraining (Chapter 4) and psychotherapy (Chapter 5).

While the neuropsychological, psychiatric, and psychosocial consequences are varied, these brain-injured patients have many problems in common. The problems that initially guided the development of the Neuropsychological Rehabilitation Program are:

Decreased motor and psychomotor functioning (to the point that gainful employment is often impossible)

Decreased speed of information-processing and possibly reduced channel capacity (dependent on perceptual and cognitive systems involved)

Variable concentration — attentional skills

Impulsiveness

Irritability and low frustration tolerance

Inappropriate social comments

Verbal expansiveness and tangential thought (possibly related to faulty feedback mechanisms)

Misperception of social comments and situations with associated problems of depression, anger, and paranoia

Eventual alienation of friends, relatives, and spouse because of inappropriate behavior with associated changes in work, marriage, and leisure activities

Unrealistic appraisal of residual neuropsychological deficits (possibly secondary to disturbances in self-awareness)

Impairment in the rate and level of new learning with associated problems of "memory" relative to psychometric intelligence

Preoccupation with how "life used to be" with associated angry outbursts, thoughts of suicide, and loss of interest and motivation in the present environment

Unrealistic expectations on the part of friends, relatives, employers, and even medical personnel because the patient frequently "looks so good" on the surface

Possible release of underlying psychiatric disturbance which was either not seen or greatly in check prior to the traumatic head injury.*

Considering these problems, and that little was being done to help those who were experiencing them, the neurosurgeons practicing at Presbyterian Hospital, along with hospital administrators, decided in 1979 to support the development of a neuropsychologically oriented treatment program

---

* This list was presented at the Traumatic Coma Data Bank Outcome Meeting, NINCDS, Bethesda, Maryland, July 25, 1980, by George P. Prigatano, Ph.D.

for young adult brain-injured patients (see Preface). Most of these patients had suffered traumatic head injury, but as indicated above, some had experienced localized cerebral anomalies as well (tumor, ruptured arteriovenous malformation, etc.). The first program began in February 1980.

Philosophy and Rationale

Rehabilitation after brain injury has historically been medically oriented. This followed logically from the need to sustain and protect an individual's life during the initial stages of recovery. Following medical stabilization, the focus was then shifted to regaining physical strength, improving ambulation, and when possible, instituting therapies to aid communication skills and help the patient become independent in basic self-care activities. The NRP approach differs in several fundamental ways from the more traditional rehabilitation setting in that it attempts to help brain-injured individuals return to a productive life-style.

First, neuropsychological deficits are seen as a primary rehabilitation target. As suggested in Chapter 4, Goldstein (1942) recognized that higher cerebral deficits needed attention in the rehabilitation of brain-injured soldiers. He suggested that such patients be given extensive psychological examinations and retrained when possible in a protected work environment. Zangwill (1947) recognized the need to remediate cognitive deficits after treating traumatic head-injury soldier patients during World War II. He discussed teaching patients compensatory techniques to get around specific higher cerebral deficits. Luria (1966) was also convinced of the need to work aggressively with higher cerebral deficits and felt that restoration of function was quite possible, particularly after focal brain damage (see Luria et al. 1969). Historically, the pioneering works of Goldstein, Zangwill, and Luria have provided the early experience and theoretical rationale for intensive cognitive-retraining activities following brain injury. In addition, Luria et al. (1969) and Ben-Yishay, Diller, and their colleagues (1970, 1971) provided practical pioneering approaches to remedy specific neuropsychological deficits.

Luria's (Luria et al. 1969) emphasis on understanding brain functions as interlocking functional subsystems has been a particularly important concept. While the diffuse and complex neuropsychological deficits that seem to accompany severe traumatic head injury make it difficult to apply Lurian assessment and remediation techniques, Luria's general approach to appreciating the interconnectedness of many cognitive functions has been vital. For example, we frequently try to teach patients how to use their existing cognitive strengths to solve an old problem that had previously been solved by other cognitive skills.

Second, in addition to addressing specific neuropsychological deficits, the NRP approach places equal emphasis on the personality of the patient and the emotional/motivational states that accompany cognitive, perceptual, motor, and language deficits (Levin and Grossman 1978) (see Chapters 3 and 5). Outcome studies following traumatic head injury emphasized that both cognitive *and* personality disturbances are related to the patient's ability to return to work and to improve interpersonal relationships (see Bond 1975; Gilchrist and Wilkinson 1979; Bruckner and Randle 1972; Walker 1972). Indeed, for some patients, personality dysfunction may overshadow cognitive deficits as the major adjustment roadblock (Fordyce et al. 1983).

Baker's (1955) work on understanding the patient's personal or intrapsychic reactions to the brain injury has helped clarify the need for psychotherapeutic interventions. Her thoughtful consideration of the patients' reactions to rehabilitation activities, including having to face the hard realities of being permanently damaged, has proven to be quite important in the clinical management of these individuals. In particular, it facilitates an analysis of patients' shame, depression, and anxiety, which time and again seem to influence their participation in an intensive rehabilitation program. Goldstein's (1942) work also helps reaffirm that some emotional and motivational disturbances may be symptoms of failing to cope and not a direct result of brain damage. Teaching patients new coping strategies, therefore, may be very therapeutic for them.

Yet there has been a pessimism among many psychotherapeutic clinicians that psychotherapy just does not work with brain-injured patients. These is some truth to this notion, if psychotherapy is undertaken in isolation from other treatments, but when integrated with the other rehabilitation activities in a consistent and intensive manner, psychotherapy in its group and individual forms provides a needed therapeutic tool with brain dysfunctional young adults (see Chapter 5).

It is our conviction that both a cognitive remediation approach and a psychotherapeutic approach to the rehabilitation of brain-injured patients, particularly traumatic head-injury patients, is needed. The NRP program considers neuropsychological rehabilitation to include both of these dimensions. In our opinion, neither is sufficient in and of itself to substantially help most brain-injured patients return to a productive life-style.

A third guiding principle of our program is that rehabilitative efforts must be intensive and integrated across rehabilitative therapies. Neuropsychological problems are frequently so disruptive to daily life that they require intensive rehabilitation efforts. Short or periodic interventions are usually not adequate. Also, because of memory deficits, patients frequently require daily practice at improving their skills. We have found that a six-month period of training is usually needed. And because brain-injured patients present with a myriad of problems and are frequently easily confused, rehabilitation themes must consistently be applied across various treatment hours. A truly integrated interdisciplinary approach is vital.

A fourth guiding principle is that rehabilitation with brain-damaged patients must constantly deal with the unrealistic appraisal patients have of their functional skills, and the patients' tendency to be unaware of or to deny residual cognitive and personality deficits (see Chapters 1, 3, and 5). At best, problems with awareness can negatively influence the patients' motivation for treatment. At worst, such problems can generate significant resistance to participating in rehabilitation activities. The important clinical issue of diminished awareness and the very closely associated phenomenon of "denial of disability" are extremely important in the psychosocial adjustment and rehabilitation of many brain-injured individuals. In the NRP a true milieu atmosphere is fostered to help address and alleviate problems of awareness and acceptance. Enhanced awareness is explicitly made a primary rehabilitation target. This is accomplished gradually and indirectly, at first with didactic educational sessions on the effects of brain injury. Later, patients are asked to record and chart their performances objectively across a variety of behavioral domains. Awareness training then becomes more directive with videotaping, public review, and the generation of individual problem lists. These lists are openly discussed and understood by all program members. Statements reflecting greater self-awareness and acceptance are rigorously reinforced by staff members and eventually by fellow patients.

Awareness and acceptance issues are also addressed in weekly relatives' meetings and in less frequent family therapy sessions. The families of brain-injured individuals may be equally unrealistic in appraising cognitive and personality deficits in their relatives (Romano 1974). In addition, it has been known for some time that relatives experience their own emotional reactions to the changes they must face with a brain-injured relative (Lezak 1978).

Selection of Patients

All patients referred for the NRP are first seen for a standardized neuropsychological examination by a clinical neuropsychologist trained in both clinical psychology and neuropsychology. All testing is done by psychologists, as opposed to technicians, since information regarding the qualitative neuropsychological responses of the patient and his or her personal reactions to testing is vital for forming some initial impressions about the suitability of the patient for intensive rehabilitative work. Patients are identified as potential candidates for the intensive Neuropsychological Rehabilitation Program based on these results, history, and interview findings. Patients typically have suffered serious brain injuries, are past the stage of rapid spontaneous recovery, and have been unable to resume a productive life-style. In nearly every case the constellation of cognitive and personality deficits forms the foundation of their adjustment problems.

Patients are not automatically accepted into the program. After the initial examination, prospective patients are seen for a series of six to eight one-hour preliminary sessions. The purpose of these sessions is to provide an initial rehabilitation trial. Information is sought regarding the following questions: How well does the patient understand his or her neuropsychological deficits? How does he or she respond to both positive and negative feedback? How unrealistic is the patient, and does this condition seem to be mediated by organic as opposed to psychiatric factors? How motivated are the patient and his or her relatives to attend sessions, keep appointments on time, and work at exercises at home? How does the patient respond to the idea of group work? What is his or her style of interpersonal interaction? What is the nature of the patient's cognitive, perceptual, motor, and language deficits?

During this time, the staff work with the patients using various cognitive remediation tasks, and their performance is explored with them and their family members. This gives the staff, the patient, and the families practical information about what goes on in an intensive rehabilitation program. It also allows all individuals involved to decide whether a six-month commitment to intensive neuropsychological rehabilitation is practical for a given individual. Information from standard neuropsychological testing that typically (but not always) rules a patient out of the program is:

IQ level below 75

WAIS or WAIS-R Digit Symbol score below 5 (usually a score of 6 or above is considered favorable, because it suggests that patients can learn at reasonable rates with repeated practice, an important skill for everyday functioning)

Wechsler Memory Quotient lower than 75

MMPI profile and/or psychiatric history suggesting psychotic disorder or severe characterological problems

Patients have to demonstrate from their history and behavior (as witnessed in the initial therapy trial and neuropsychological examination) a basic ability to talk about painful issues and the motivation to engage in rehabilitation activities. Repeated failure to keep appointments and/or an inability to engage in basic cognitive retraining and psychotherapeutic tasks would exclude a patient. Finally, a commitment by the family to involve themselves in the rehabilitation program as deemed necessary is highly desirable and in some instances absolutely necessary. Without family participation, generalization of progress made during rehabilitation to home environments becomes unlikely.

Patients involved in the NRP to date have been varied in terms of the degree of neuropsychological impairment. Most have had traumatic head injuries, but a number have had localized lesions. The degree of long-term residual neuropsychological impairment has varied from mild to severe, as indicated by the Average Impairment Rating (see Prigatano, Fordyce et al. 1983). Most patients are nonaphasic, but three aphasic patients have been treated in our program. All these patients had the basic ability to comprehend at least functionally what was said to them. All have been able to care for personal hygiene needs and have been ambulatory with at least the use of a cane. Some patients, however, have been clearly amnestic, but they retained other cognitive skills that could be the basis for a retraining program.

The Program

The general format of the Neuropsychological Rehabilitation Program is a structured outpatient day-treatment program. The rehabilitation day is broken up into formally differentiated treatment hours (lasting fifty minutes). The morning sessions occur in group format, while the afternoon sessions are individually delivered, with the exception of the final session of each treatment day. Patients are worked with for approximately six hours a day, four days a week for six months. Six to eight patients are worked with by five to six therapists: three clinical neuropsychologists, one speech and language pathologist, one occupational therapist, and one physical therapist.

9:00–9:50 A.M., COGNITIVE RETRAINING

While the variability in specific neuropsychological deficits following brain injury is large, some general processes are likely to be disrupted (see Chapter 1). These include attentional deficits, perceptual dysfunction, learning and memory disorders, reduced abstraction skills, reduced problem-solving skills, and slowed basic information-processing speed (e.g., Bond 1975; Goldstein 1942; Gronwall and Sampson 1974; Levin et al. 1979; Mandleberg and Brooks 1975). Cognitive retraining, occurring during the first hour of each treatment day, addresses these general cognitive deficits.

Two to three patients work with a single staff member (a clinical psychologist, an occupational therapist, or a speech and language pathologist) on a system of hierarchically arranged paper-and-pencil cognitive tasks. The task content is basic at first, involving simple fine-motor speed and basic orientation. As performance improves and asymptotes, more complex tasks are added and simple ones are dropped. Daily scores and times are recorded for each patient in individual notebooks, and once a week average weekly scores are graphed. While these activities occur in a group format, each patient moves through the tasks at his or her own rate of speed.

The staff first monitor the patients' behavior and then have the patients monitor their performance on the same tasks. This allows the patients to see that the staff is willing to expose their cognitive strengths and weaknesses. It also allows the patients to compare their performances with that of non-brain-damaged individuals as well as with those of fellow patients. This allows for growing awareness of strengths and weaknesses in a non-threatening small-group (or dyad) situation. Within this general context, several specific goals are pursued:

1. Patients are trained to use problem-solving skills that focus on the use of strategies. The daily graphing of progress without strategies, with poor or inefficient strategies, and finally with good strategies results in a stressing of the practical benefits of strategies and/or compensations without placing the therapist in the role of lecturer. By comparing daily scores and weekly graphs, patients discover for themselves the effects of strategies and are less resistant to their use. This technique may also be used to convince some patients that they frequently may not be able to come up with strategies on their own and will have to rely on others to provide a template for their own problem-solving.

2. Patients compile objective evidence of their performance to help increase their awareness of their strengths and deficits. The weekly graphing of performance and daily recording of scores for use *by the patient* serves to provide an objective quantified number to some of the patients' behaviors. For patients who are not aware of deficits, numbers lower than those of other patients working at the same table bring home the point without the staff's being the sole bearer of bad news. For patients who are excessively depressed over the effects of brain injury, increasing scores are brought up as evidence of improvement. It is much more difficult for a patient to say that hard numbers are "just someone else's opinion that I am improving."

3. Patients' ability to calculate, graph, and record is determined. Patients frequently evidence confusion, memory problems, calculation problems, and slowness in recording and graphing. Since recording is a real-life task with benefits that the patient can recognize, it is treated as a problem to be solved. Such solutions as the use of electronic pocket calculators, verbal compensations for memory loss by asking others for information, and referring to a written list of procedures are used. The patient learns that compensations are a form of strategy.

4. Information about performance in this hour is used to guide other treatment activities for the patients. The integrated daily use of informa-

tion derived in one hour to guide therapy in a different hour is a major point of difference between this program and traditional rehabilitation team approaches.

5. Patients' work performance characteristics are assessed. A patient can usually be shown in an immediate and practical manner the effects of fatigue, rest breaks, and conversational distraction on his or her performance of a well-routinized behavior. These characteristics will then be incorporated in vocational planning or may be modified with training during the patient's individual cognitive retraining hour.

10:00–10:50 A.M., COGNITIVE GROUP THERAPY

The second hour of each treatment day has two major goals. The first is to identify and remediate residual cognitive deficits as they are reflected in the thinking and communication difficulties of individual patients. The second is to directly facilitate increased self-awareness of residual deficits and current strengths. Both goals are accomplished in a group therapy format led by a clinical neuropsychologist and a speech and language pathologist. All rehabilitation patients are present.

With respect to the remediation of cognitive deficits, initial emphasis is placed on identification of specific problems in thinking and communication which are common following brain injury. A formal simplified system is presented, describing traditional aphasic problems, nonaphasic communication disorders, and cognitive disorders that accompany brain injury (Prigatano et al. in press). Each patient is helped to understand his or her particular difficulties. There is heavy emphasis on the more common nonaphasic communication problems and related cognitive difficulties, because they tend to be more subtle and less easily identified. These include the tendency to talk excessively, to become tangential in communication (i.e., wandering from one topic to the next), to interrupt ongoing conversation, to forget the topic of conversation, to speak inappropriately with potentially offensive results, and to employ peculiar words and phraseology during conversation. Such difficulties are frequently associated with problems of inattention, impulsivity, "concrete" thinking, and memory dysfunction.

As these ideas are presented to patients and rehearsed, each patient is slowly brought to the point of being able to understand how his or her own brain injury has affected the ability to interact cognitively in social environments. As awareness and acceptance are slowly accomplished, compensation strategies and techniques designed to offset these difficulties are introduced. These are subsequently practiced and monitored informally in highly structured group activities and formally in specific role-playing exercises. Videotape is used extensively as the program progresses and the patient is able to tolerate such direct feedback. This helps patients evaluate the impact compensations have on thinking and communication effectiveness. Toward the end of the program, the communication situations practiced in the group become more complex and more lifelike. Conflict resolution, dating, explaining the injury to others, interpersonal interaction, job interviews, and other practically oriented role-playing scenarios are designed and rehearsed to help patients deal effectively with the inevitable stresses encountered in the transition to productive living.

Facilitation of self-awareness begins after a sense of comfortableness and trust has developed between patients and staff. Exercises are systematized and gradually introduced to inhibit catastrophic reactions, denial, and defensiveness. Initially, problems in awareness are discussed impersonally through previous case examples, including the review of videotapes of earlier patients. Subsequently, a model of the stages of recovery following brain injury is presented and discussed. This model emphasizes issues of awareness and acceptance of residual deficits and has been developed by our staff to facilitate awareness training. Through a large flowchart mounted permanently on the treatment room wall, this model takes a typical closed-head-injury patient from the time of injury through the stages of coma and intensive care, posttraumatic amnesia, acute rehabilitation, medical discharge, and problems in returning to the old way of life. Efforts are made to show how cognitive/communication problems and the incomplete awareness or tendency to deny problems can create predictable emotional, interpersonal, and vocational problems at each stage of recovery. Each patient attempts to identify the state of recovery in which he or she is currently. Group members, in turn, give the patient public feedback as to the accuracy of their choice. This process of contrasting group and individual opinion frequently provides the first clear evidence that individual patients may be perceiving themselves differently from the way others see them. Finally, patients are videotaped, and the videotape is reviewed specifically to identify current strengths and weaknesses. Patients initially attempt to review their own tapes. This is followed by group feedback and formal discussion. The result is a public list of strengths and weaknesses which serves as a foundation for a problem list for each patient, posted on the treatment room wall. Each list contains the cognitive and personality problems that staff and patient agree are critical to the person's successful rehabilitation.

The process of facilitating awareness and acceptance is a delicate one. Therapists must be sensitive to the emotional and motivational state of each patient. In particular, each patient's ability to tolerate critical feedback has to be clinically assessed. Objective impartial evidence is utilized as much as possible, and the identification of weaknesses is balanced aggressively with the identification of realistic strengths. Statements that show awareness of or acceptance of residual problems, or obvious indications of conscious appropriate compensation for residual problems, receive intensive public reinforcement. Throughout the course of cognitive group therapy, progress in the specific problems in thinking, of communication, and of awareness and acceptance are repeatedly reviewed and, when possible, recorded and graphed. Earlier videotapes are saved and compared with tapes made at the end of therapy to capture for each patient the improvements, or lack thereof, over the course of cognitive group therapy.

A Clinical Example of Cognitive Group Therapy

To highlight how cognitive group therapy actually works in practice, a detailed clinical example is provided here. The example focuses on helping disinhibited patients to be more socially appropriate in their comments and more clear and concise in what they say. These two problems, social inappropriateness and tangentiality of language, seem to be related to the neuropsychological deficits of these patients. In the context of cognitive group therapy, a frequent scenario is as follows:

One of the therapists asks the patients to introduce themselves. The patients may begin by stating their names and the fact that they had an accident. From there comments typically wander, and they get off the topic. For example, when hypothetical patient Joe is asked, "Why are you here?" he states that he was in an automobile accident and suffered a brain injury. Then he says that he was driving a Chevy down highway I-40 and that the Chevy was a 1980 model. He then states that his aunt in Wisconsin has a Chevy of similar vintage. From there he wanders to say that the aunt also has a farm and raises bulls, and then he begins to discuss the question of how bulls are bred. At this point the therapist interrupts and points out to Joe that he has greatly strayed from the topic. The therapist then asks whether any of the other patients in the group experience these difficulties. As is frequently the case, no one admits to these problems, and some of the patients might even criticize the therapist for being too picky in his or her observations. The therapist then asks the patients to participate in the following exercise: Patients are asked to introduce themselves again and to describe what they do, but this time the therapist chooses a second patient, for example, hypothetical patient John, to monitor the verbalizations of Joe. The therapist asks John to raise his hand when Joe begins to stray from the topic. This is attempted, and as is typically the case, John does not raise his hand when Joe becomes tangential. At this point the therapist, in a very animated way, may interrupt and state that the patient has, in fact, just gotten off the track. A discussion usually ensues as to whose observations are right and whose are wrong. At this point the therapist introduces the concept of a videotape to provide an objective measure of how clear a patient's communication is and to show exactly when the patient begins to stray from the topic. The therapist and patients are now working more as allies, attempting to find some objective record of when a failure in communication occurs.

Once the videotape is introduced, the therapist can begin to go back with patients and show them how they get off the topic. This procedure allows the therapist to avoid criticizing the patient directly but to state objectively that there is a problem of tangentiality in comments. Patients can see that they vary in the degree to which they have this problem and often can see the problems in others before they can see them in themselves. This is an extremely important point that is made in cognitive group therapy. Patients are asked to identify the communication difficulties of other patients and then to see the degree to which these problems apply to themselves. This type of didactic procedure is very helpful in that it does not criticize the patients but brings home the point that there are failures in communication they may not be aware of.

The same type of thing can occur for socially inappropriate comments or behaviors. For example, one patient may smile or laugh when talking about something that is painful or distressing. Patients who make these inappropriate comments or reactions may not be aware of their impact on others. Again, by videotaping them during such sessions, patients can see firsthand how they are responding inappropriately and what reactions others are having. This type of feedback provides the objective record that is often necessary in order to bring home to a patient problems in responsiveness in social interaction which cause major interpersonal difficulties.

The cognitive group therapy hour was specifically designed for these types of problems. The focus is on problems that clearly have a cognitive basis to them and therefore are more directly related to the degree and type of cerebral dysfunction.

11:00-11:50 A.M., GROUP PSYCHOTHERAPY

After the more cognitively oriented group activities, patients are seen in group psychotherapy, which is conducted by two psychologists who are trained in both clinical psychology and neuropsychology. The focus is on the emotional and motivational difficulties frequently associated with brain damage. Problems dealing primarily with the catastrophic reaction and premorbid personality characteristics, which influence rehabilitation activities, are discussed. However, neuropsychological and personality disturbances are also discussed, and the patients are given a mini-course in the neurology and neuropsychology of their brain injury.

Each group psychotherapy hour begins with an identification by a group member of the name of the hour, its purpose, and why it is an important part of the rehabilitation program. Patients are taught that the purpose of the hour is to "discuss feelings and emotions." This is important, because "how you feel determines how you act" and "how you act determines how other people react to you." The point is made that frequently after brain injury people experience negative reactions from others that they do not fully understand and that group psychotherapy should help them in this regard. It is also pointed out that many people believe it is a waste of time to try to do psychotherapy with brain-injured patients. The reasons behind this are given: problems in paying attention, memory, and understanding what is said may make psychotherapy useless with brain-injured patients. A fourth point is that after brain injury there may be less control over one's affective reactions, and some are concerned that brain-injured people will only get more upset after discussing painful topics. It is pointed out that if patients can compensate for these four problems, they can benefit from a discussion of personality difficulties. It is also pointed out that brain injury does not wipe out one's humanness, or the need to have an integrated sense of self. Consequently, it is argued, group psychotherapy is a major part of a rehabilitation program if an individual is going to reestablish a sense of identity and begin to integrate his or her life.

Early in treatment, patients are asked to address specific questions concerning their personality functioning as they presently perceive it. They are asked to identify which emotional and motivational problems they have experienced in themselves since their injury. Then, they are asked to document their relatives' perceptions of their personality difficulties. This process is facilitated by introducing and reviewing a formal list of affective problems that have been associated with brain injury. In a sense, this provides a menu of personality difficulties from which the patient can pick and choose, reflecting what the patient experiences or what relatives think he or she has experienced. The concept of the catastrophic reaction is gently woven into this initial discussion.

Since one of the psychotherapists leading the group psychotherapy session is also a co-leader of the cognitive group therapy, transfer of emotional and motivational topics generated in the cognitive group to the group psychotherapy session is facilitated. When the patient becomes angry, upset, or depressed during cognitive group therapy, he or she is told that this can be discussed within the context of group psychotherapy, which will occur shortly. This teaches the patient the importance of control and of bringing up affective issues at the appropriate time. It also fosters a recognition by all therapists that there are inevitably emotional and motivational difficulties which should be formally addressed.

Group psychotherapy activities then focus on the neuropsychologically based personality disturbances. Patients are taught as much about the brain and their unique brain injuries as possible. This is a didactic portion of the group psychotherapy hour and strays furthest from the more traditional psychiatric group psychotherapy format. Yet it provides valuable insights for patients as they learn to understand their behavior by understanding their neuropsychological disturbances. A brief and simplified overview of functional neuroanatomy is presented, employing films, slides, videotapes, and models of the brain. Each patient's medical history, x-rays, and CT scans are obtained, and appropriate slides are made. This information is reviewed and discussed publicly from the standpoint of helping the patients understand how their cognitive and affective problems have come about. This also helps other patients become more empathetic toward each other, since they now recognize that some personality disturbances may be as organically mediated as a hemiparesis or an aphasic disturbance. The amount and pace of this didactic information is dictated by the amount of information the patients can process as well as the overall tone that exists in a typical rehabilitation day. When there is a lot of tension, we have found that discussion of this more "intellectual" material helps settle everyone down. We also found that this didactic information conveys to the patients the notion that even though they are brain-damaged they can still learn important information about themselves. This strengthens their self-esteem and gives them a new feeling of dignity about themselves as individuals. It also fosters a true milieu experience.

The next formal section of psychotherapy involves discussion of the premorbid personality characteristics of characterological problems that may have anteceded the injury. The purpose of this discussion is to demonstrate to patients how their brain injury interacts with previous characteristics to determine their current constellation of strengths and weaknesses. This particular activity typically meets with the greatest resistance among the rehabilitation patients. If these premorbid personality traits are not understood and dealt with, however, the patient will just repeat many of the psychosocial problems, in an exaggerated fashion, that they had prior to the injury. We have found that the use of humor and reference to published scientific work helps patients talk about premorbid difficulties. This provides for a nonthreatening but realistic discussion of how each patient's personality may be contributing to his or her own failures in adapting or, conversely, may be helping him or her adapt. These usually powerful discussions help the patients take personal responsibility for what is happening to them.

Problems with parents, spouses, children, and friends are also discussed within the context of a neuropsychological, behavioral, and psychodynamic perspective. The patients are encouraged to look at what practical steps they can take to enhance their ability to get along with others and to maintain satisfactory interpersonal relationships.

Finally, toward the end of the six months, group psychotherapy patients are asked to function in a more traditional psychiatric manner. Group leaders say relatively little, but try to facilitate discussions with patients. The purpose is to see the degree to which the individual can listen to and interact with others in an unstructured environment using emotionally and interpersonally appropriate behaviors. If the patients are able to deal with this type of unstructured activity without losing emotional control, it is a reasonably good sign of more effective interpersonal adjustment.

1:00–1:50 P.M. AND 2:00–2:50 P.M., INDIVIDUAL THERAPY

After lunch, each patient receives two separate sessions of individual therapy. This may include some combination of individual psychotherapy, speech and language therapy, occupational therapy, cognitive retraining, physical therapy, or vocational counseling and placement activities. On the basis of initial evaluations, the individual problems the patient experiences are identified, and these are addressed in these individual hours. With the exception of psychotherapy, which every patient receives, the nature of the particular individual therapies depends on a patient's particular problems. A patient's schedule of afternoon activities may also change over the course of rehabilitation.

The cognitive retraining tasks given during this individualized time are not repetitions of the simplified speed of information-processing tasks given in the morning hour. These modules are integrated forms of problem-solving and skill remediation. For example, if the patient presents a visuospatial deficit, this may initially be retrained through the use of verbal descriptions of geometric materials to solve visuospatial problems. Later training may include teaching the rules of gestalt (proximity, closure, similarity, continuity) to facilitate visual-spatial problem-solving skills directly. The retraining progressively becomes integrated into vocational planning (e.g., map reading, taking bus routes, manual work on materials with many angles, operating equipment). Finally, the effects of the patient's deficits are determined and minimized in simulated work settings. Cognitive, perceptual, language, or motor deficits that are to be remediated are approached in a similar manner. The goal is to facilitate as close an approximation to normal, independent life skills and vocational functioning as possible.

An Example of Individual Cognitive Retraining

As the name implies, the individual forms of cognitive retraining are quite variable and depend on the specific problems that a given patient has. Frequently, the patients who have suffered frontal lobe injuries have a series of cognitive deficits that make them much less socially acceptable and greatly enhance their psychosocial difficulties. While there is no prototype for doing cognitive retraining on an individual basis, it is hoped that the following example will be of use to therapists in the field and give some indication of what is actually done within the context of our neuropsychological rehabilitation program.

The patient to be discussed is a young man who was injured in a small-plane crash. (He is not the one referred to earlier.) This patient initially did not recognize any neuropsychological sequelae from his injury. Moreover, when his wife would report that he did not seem to take things seriously, he would frequently smile or make inane comments. Eventually his wife became so frustrated that she left him. With this, he felt that entering the Neuropsychological Rehabilitation Program might result in his wife's returning to him, so he returned for treatment and was seen within the context of the entire program. The speech and language pathologist who worked with him in cognitive group therapy recognized that this man needed individual time to identify specifically the socially inappropriate behaviors that seemed to be a result of his brain injury and/or premorbid personality characteristics. By using the background of group work, as well as general feedback on how the patient was doing in the program, a list of socially inappropriate, irritating behaviors could be compiled. The therapist and the patient worked together to construct this list, although the therapist did the bulk of work. The list developed was as follows:

1. A tendency to provide lip service when about to make impulsive or inappropriate statements. For example, there is a tendency to say "I know this is impulsive" or "I know this is going to be inappropriate" and then to go ahead and make statements that fit in that category.
2. A tendency to make unrealistic statements regarding the program or the staff. Statements such as "This is the best program in the world" or "You guys are fantastic and incredibly great" are frequently made, even when the patient appears at times to be uncooperative and antagonistic.
3. A tendency to pay excessive attention to certain female patients who are uncomfortable with that attention and to warn female patients that he may be dangerous, which obviously would upset them.
4. A tendency to give the impression to others that negative feedback is taken with a grain of salt and that nothing seems to get through. This frequently results in others becoming angry or frustrated with the patient.
5. A tendency to make comments that suggest that the patient has superiority over others or at least intellectual superiority. Again this tends to alienate others.
6. A tendency to answer questions with a question, as opposed to making a direct or positive comment.
7. A tendency to wink at others and say "Yes ma'am" or "Yes sir" when

talking to staff or fellow patients when they make critical comments to the patient.

All these behaviors were specifically listed as socially inappropriate and irritating. The list was developed on a one-to-one basis, that is, with one therapist and one patient, so that the patient could come to grips with the specifics of what he was doing that was causing trouble in his rehabilitation.

After this list was constructed, within the confines of individual cognitive retraining, a specific set of alternative behaviors was devised and agreed on between the therapist and the patient. Those suggested alternative behaviors were as follows:

1. Be more direct in expressing opinions or thoughts, without prefacing statements that allude to inappropriateness, poor judgment, or impulsivity.
2. Generate a list of appropriate comments that you may make to other members of the program, staff, or the program itself.
3. Discuss in group psychotherapy underlying feelings or fantasies that underpin desires to have contact with a specific female patient, rather than showing excessive interest in female patients during the program.
4. Develop a more serious attitude to the rehabilitation process as a whole.
5. Begin to explore what are reasonable reactions to painful feedback or difficult issues being raised in reference to you.
6. Develop a better understanding of the intellectual deficits that are directly related to your brain damage.
7. Develop a more direct style of expressing opinions or providing examples, one which utilizes a feeling of honesty and directness rather than superiority.

By going over these individual dimensions, the patient and therapist could devise a strategy that the individual could adopt and utilize throughout the rehabilitation day. This one-on-one interaction was necessary in order for the patients to figure out how to start to deal with others more appropriately within the context of the group program. It was also pointed out that many of these socially inappropriate and irritating behaviors stem directly from the brain damage. The patient could progressively come to grips with this and utilize different behavioral strategies for coping with them. This is an example of how dealing with the cognitive underpinnings of a neuropsychologically based personality-psychosocial problem can have substantial impact on at least the patient's eventual sociability. More work of this type is needed, and the whole field of individual cognitive retraining, as previously mentioned, is in its infancy.

3:00–3:45 P.M., INDEPENDENT SUPERVISED THERAPY

The purpose of the hour for independent supervised therapy is to help foster independence and the individual patient's capacity to work productively under minimal supervision. Each patient is asked to work relatively independently for this forty-five-minute period several times each week. Initially, structure is provided in the form of particular assignments, which are discussed in individual therapy sessions. Later, patients are encouraged to become more independent, and the degree of structure and supervision is reduced. To the extent that patients can manage increased autonomy during this time, they are more ready to undertake work situations in the real world.

3:45–4:15 P.M., MILIEU

The final treatment session of the day involves a meeting of the entire rehabilitation community, including all patients and all staff members. This time provides an opportunity for brief discussion of rehabilitation issues before the entire community. Important rehabilitation events, positive or negative, that occurred during the day are reviewed and briefly discussed. Any business items related to the smooth running of the program are also discussed during milieu. Thus, the milieu hour helps promote the continuity and consistency which is so important in rehabilitating brain-injured individuals.

4:30–5:15 P.M., STAFF MEETING*

Following milieu, the treatment staff has its daily meeting. Documentation and accounting work are briefly done for each rehabilitation day. Then the progress of each patient for that particular rehabilitation day is reviewed, possible changes in intervention are discussed, and staff members are generally kept abreast of the patient's performance. When particularly critical or sensitive therapeutic issues arise, as is inevitable for each patient, the staff collectively and carefully plan the most productive strategy for dealing with these issues. This ensures that patients receive a consistent therapeutic theme on a daily basis. It also allows the staff to capitalize on their own therapeutic strengths rather than attempting to manage unfamiliar or uncomfortable situations in a less produtive manner. In addition to these important clinical activities, the daily staff meeting serves another vital purpose. It provides a chance for staff members to give each other support, guidance, and a productive outlet for the frustrations that naturally develop when working so closely with patients. We have dis-

---

*On Wednesdays, the Staff Meeting adjourns at 5:00 P.M. so that staff members can conduct the Relatives' Group.

covered that without such an opportunity, the tremendous commitment of staff energy required by such an intensive program can be overwhelming.

5:00–6:00 P.M., WEDNESDAY NIGHTS, RELATIVES' GROUP

Once a week the primary relatives of patients involved in the rehabilitation program meet for an hourly session. This session is usually conducted by two of the staff psychologists. At various times, however, all rehabilitation staff members rotate into this meeting, to provide an opportunity for mutual exchange with relatives. These weekly meetings with relatives have two major purposes. First, they provide a forum for the mutual exchange of information concerning the patient's behavior at home and in the program, they provide an opportunity for staff members to give each relative the details of major treatment strategies and progress, and they allow staff members to hear what difficulties continue to occur at home and to offer suggestions as to how they might be handled. Second, Relatives' Group provides an important emotional outlet for the people living with our brain-injured patients. The pain and frustration incurred by the relatives of brain-injured individuals are well known (Lezak 1978), and this population certainly benefits from supportive counseling sessions. In our experience, the group format provides a powerful means by which relatives can educate and support each other.

In addition to these weekly relatives' meetings, episodic individual family counseling sessions are also scheduled as needed. In particular, husband-wife dyads that experience a great deal of marital stress are met with more frequently in family counseling sessions by one or two staff members. While the major focus of our program is to make the brain-injured individual more productive and independent, this cannot occur in isolation. The social environment must be considered and worked with.

Medical Consultants

The staff meet monthly with an experienced psychiatrist to discuss the management of various patients and their families. This has proven to be helpful in getting a perspective that cannot be had from within the program. In addition, other psychiatrists are contacted to help with patient medication needs on a routine basis.

The initial physical examination is usually accomplished by the referring physicians (typically neurosurgeons and/or neurologists). When other medical consultation is needed, it is done through the referring physician.

Staff Development and Interdisciplinary Staff Relationships

Intensive work with brain-injured patients is a difficult task for even the most capable therapists. Brain injury produces a myriad of problems, many of which are permanent or very slow to change. Staff members can become confused, frustrated, and fatigued, just like patients and their families. They need support, continuing education, and relief from this type of work if they are to remain energetic and dedicated to the treatment task. Conducting the rehabilitation program Monday through Thursday helps give staff members a break from the extensive work schedule. On Fridays, they typically see patients not in the program or engage in research and educational activities.

While many decisions regarding patients are truly group decisions, staff members also need a leader. Unless someone takes clinical responsibility for integrating treatment approaches and clarifying treatment issues, the staff do not have the structure and support they need to carry out their mission. The group leader need not come from any one discipline, but he or she should clearly be identified as the most experienced and knowledgeable individual in that particular group when it comes to working with the patients.

Staff members also need an opportunity for meaningful continued education. A tremendous amount of information is available regarding brain-behavior relationships and their disturbances after brain injury. There is also a good deal of information regarding the emotional/motivational problems of these patients. No single discipline has the market on the truth when it comes to rehabilitating brain-injured patients. Consequently, staff members need to be exposed to wide sources of information in order to continue to be effective with these patients and remain energetic and thoughtful about their work. This exposure should come in the form of presenting old as well as new ideas pertinent to the rehabilitation process.

Staff members need a time to express their frustration and irritation with patients as well as with one another. When the clinical work does not go well, staff members can become easily irritated with the patients, and this can influence their relationship with other staff members. A format for dealing with this irritation within the context of staff meetings is vital. If this is not present, then interdisciplinary staff feuds can develop, job satisfaction can decrease, and turnover can be high.

Initial Impressions and Ideas Concerning Outcome Measures

The next chapter will deal formally with the outcome findings of the Neuropsychological Rehabilitation Program, but here we note some initial impressions that may be clinically relevant and that helped guide our understanding as to what one should measure as appropriate outcome indices.

The basic questions regarding intensive neuropsychological rehabilitation are: Can the rate or level of neuropsychological functioning be improved after brain injury using various forms of cognitive remediation? Can personality difficulties be substantially altered by the combination of cognitive retraining and psychotherapy? Can patients be trained to return to a productive life-style? And is such training cost-efficient?

It has been our impression that modest improvement of neuropsychological functioning is possible with extensive retraining past the period of spontaneous recovery (see Prigatano et al. 1984), but the amount of improvement appears to be relatively small. Consequently, it may be more productive to teach the patients to become aware of their deficits and find ways to compensate for them than to hope for substantial change in neuropsychological status. More data is needed to answer the question as to what ultimate level of neuropsychological recovery is possible. At this point, however, we would agree with Zangwill's (1947) observations that teaching compensation techniques may be the most expeditious way of training such individuals.

Personality disturbances that are part of the catastrophic reaction following brain injury can be substantially modified. They are, in our experience, clearly tied to rehabilitation success (i.e., the ability of the patient to maintain employment). This has been documented elsewhere (Prigatano et al. 1984). Suffice it to say that cognitive deficits are not as important as personality disturbances in predicting eventual recovery in this patient population once minimum cognitive skills are obtained (e.g., IQ greater than 75). We have data to suggest that when patients become belligerent, helpless, and unwilling to accept what has happened to them, they have the poorest work adjustment. Recent data also suggest that without active intervention personality difficulties may enhance with the passage of time rather than spontaneously improve (Fordyce et al. 1983).

Some chronic unemployed brain-injured patients certainly can be helped to be returned to gainful employment, but the process is difficult and the parameters for predicting successful readjustment are not easy to define. Basically, however, we have been convinced that at least low-average IQ and the ability to compensate for memory, perceptual, and motor deficits are vital. We also are convinced that the presence of a psychotic disturbance or severe characterological problem is a stronger predictor of failure. Patients who can become aware of their difficulties, accept those difficulties, and lower their sights to more realistic goals make the best success. While we have attempted to correlate the locus and type of lesion with eventual recovery, we have worked with too few patients to make any definitive statements in this regard. However, it is our present clinical impression that patients with extensive temporal lobe disturbances can be the most difficult to rehabilitate. They tend to be easily angered, paranoid, and unrealistic in their self-appraisal. Their cognitive deficits are also substantial. In contrast, patients who have mainly frontal lobe injuries are often more amenable to this form of rehabilitation. Their unawareness of deficit seems to be organically mediated, and with daily feedback they are able to change their perceptions more easily. They are less suspicious and less complicated in their cognitive deficits.

Reliable statistics on the percentage of patients who are able to get back to gainful employment after traumatic head injury are not available. From the few studies in the literature, it appears that perhaps only one-third of severe head-injury patients (i.e., those who are in a coma for at least twenty-four hours) are able to return to gainful employment through the traditional rehabilitative efforts. In the first eighteen traumatic head-injury patients who have gone through our program, approximately 50 to 60 percent of the patients have been able to obtain and maintain employment. We are hopeful that, with refined selection criteria, this figure may eventually be moved up to 75 percent.

Finally, the question of cost-efficiency of this and other programs must be seriously considered. The NRP, as a day treatment program, requires less nonessential staff time and more modest facilities compared with inpatient rehabilitation facilities. Patient fees range from $15,000 to $20,000 per patient per six-month program. While this is a substantial figure, it is considerably less than the cost of inpatient rehabilitation. Program fees must reflect the costs of operation (primarily the salaries of staff members), the local economic conditions, the ability of third-party payors to authorize such treatment, and so on. We have found this figure to be acceptable to many of the parties involved in providing the funds for this form of rehabilitation. We are presently considering alternate ways of streamlining our program to make it even more cost-efficient. This is a difficult venture, but one that is necessary if neuropsychological rehabilitative programs are to survive the fiscal realities of life.

The question of what are adequate outcome measures is always a difficult one to answer. The percentage of patients who are able to return to gainful employment has to be the most important criterion. From society's perspective, these successes will not only prove to be less of an economic burden, because of the reduction in disability benefits, but also become taxpayers. If the patients who are rehabilitated are able to pay taxes, then one can demonstrate that they are ultimately able to contribute finances to the very system which initially sponsored their rehabilitation. If this takes place, we will have a system that supports itself.

A third outcome measure centers on the quality of life that the patients and their families have. The degree of marital adjustment, the capacity to tolerate the normal stresses of life, and the feelings of belonging and well-being are important indices of overall outcome. While such measures are important from a social and humanistic point of view, they are not weighed heavily by agencies that must pay for the cost of these treatments.

In this regard, it is interesting to note that of all the research that has been done on the effectiveness of psychotherapy, nothing has supported its economic continuance more than research that has been carried out in health maintenance organizations (HMOs). In HMOs it has been shown that psychotherapy substantially reduces the use of other expensive medical procedures, and consequently it has been supported within such systems (Cummings 1977). It may well be that the ultimate effectiveness of neuropsychological rehabilitation programs will be judged on these same criteria. What reduction in cost accrues to insurance companies or state and federal agencies by having the patient in an intensive neuropsychological rehabilitation program? Does the patient make less-frequent visits to neurosurgeons, neurologists, or interns? Does the patient need less medication, fewer repeat EEGs and CT scans, and so on? Do patients and their families require less consultation time with psychiatrists? Is there a lower rate of alcoholism, divorce, and job turnover? These social and economic questions should be addressed in any comprehensive outcome study.

Summary

The Neuropsychological Rehabilitation Program at Presbyterian Hospital in Oklahoma City was developed in response to the need to help young adult brain-injured patients return to productive living when traditional rehabilitation efforts were inadequate. The program, which began in February 1980, draws heavily on the earlier work of Goldstein, Zangwill, Luria, and Baker and the present work of Ben-Yishay. It is unique insofar as it fosters *both* cognitive retraining and a psychotherapeutic approach to neuropsychological rehabilitation. Small groups of patients are worked with intensively, four days a week, six hours a day, for six months by an interdisciplinary team of three clinical neuropsychologists, one speech and language pathologist, one occupational therapist, and two part-time physical therapists. Both individual and group exercises are followed in a fairly structured routine. Patients are helped to become aware of their residual cognitive and personality strengths and weaknesses. They are helped to remediate and compensate for these deficits. The importance of an integrated treatment effort by all staff members is emphasized.

CHAPTER 7
The Outcome of Neuropsychological Rehabilitation Efforts

George P. Prigatano, David J. Fordyce, Harriet K. Zeiner, James R. Roueche, Mary Pepping, and Beth Case Wood

Assessing the effectiveness of the Neuropsychological Rehabilitation Program at Presbyterian Hospital in Oklahoma City has been an ongoing research and clinical venture since its inception. In this chapter, the initial outcome data on eighteen closed-head-injury patients seen for such intensive neuropsychologically oriented rehabilitation are presented. In addition, seventeen closed-head-injury patients who underwent traditional rehabilitation, but for one reason or another were unable to undergo intensive cognitive retraining and psychotherapeutic rehabilitation, served as controls. Both sets of patients were referred for neuropsychological assessment, and both sets were deemed to need intensive rehabilitation above and beyond traditional means. Data were obtained regarding neuropsychological functioning, personality characteristics, and psychosocial adjustment (particularly work adjustment). In addition, the characteristics of those patients who were successful in returning to a productive life-style were compared with those of NRP patients who did not return to work.

While adequate outcome statistics are not available, present estimates suggest that only one-third of severe closed-head-injury patients may be helped to return to gainful employment using traditional rehabilitation methods (Weddell et al. 1980; Gilchrist and Wilkinson 1979). A large number of these unemployed patients literally walk and talk, but they experience significant difficulties in returning to work and establishing interpersonal relationships. While the purpose of this initial outcome study was to determine whether there was any significant change in neuropsychological and personality functioning, the major question was whether these patients could substantially be returned to a more productive life-style than what had been accomplished by traditional means. It has been the ratio-

---

An earlier version of this chapter appeared in *Journal of Neurology, Neurosurgery, and Psychiatry*, 1984, *47*, 505–513.

nale of our Neuropsychological Rehabilitation Program that a combination of cognitive retraining and psychotherapy would be necessary to accomplish these goals. With this in mind, these patients were selected, treated, and studied to determine the effectiveness of the NRP as it presently exists.

Subjects

Patients seen in Neuropsychological Rehabilitation Program at Presbyterian Hospital came from a larger population of outpatient referrals for neuropsychological evaluation following serious brain injury. Between February 1980 and August 1982, twenty-eight patients accepted the recommendation for participation in the NRP and entered the program. Of these twenty-eight patients, twenty-two had suffered significant traumatic head injury. Four of these twenty-two traumatic head-injury patients dropped out of the program before completion and were excluded from analysis in the present investigation. This left a core population of eighteen traumatic head-injury patients who completed at least six months of work in the NRP. Three of these patients were seen for an additional six-month term in the NRP, but analyses of improvements in neuropsychological test data are based on only the first six-month program for these subjects. The general characteristics of this population of eighteen head-injury patients are shown in Table 7.1. Virtually all of them had cerebral contusions and/or brain-stem contusion. As a group, patients were past the period of rapid spontaneous recovery (Bond 1975), with a mean chronicity of 21.6 months. Three had a posttraumatic seizure disorder, twelve had residual paresis, and six had residual signs of aphasia and/or dysarthria. All patients experienced substantial problems in postinjury adjustment.

From the same neuropsychological referral population from which the NRP patients originated, a group of similar traumatic head-injury patients was selected to serve as controls. All neuropsychological test files for traumatic head-injury patients seen between February 1980 and August 1982 were retrospectively examined. The initial selection was a function of how closely each potential control patient matched the age, sex, education level, injury severity (as measured by the Russell-Neuringer Average Impairment Rating) (Prigatano, Parsons et al. 1983), and time-since-injury characteristics of the NRP patients. From this group of subjects, seventeen controls were culled on the basis of having a subsequent follow-up neuropsychological examination at a time interval that approximated the interest interval of the NRP patients. The variables of age, sex, education level, injury severity, and chronicity have all been shown to influence either outcome following brain injury or neuropsychological test performance (Bond and Brooks 1976; Fordyce et al. 1983; Braakman et al. 1980; Jennett et al. 1977; Lewin et al. 1979; Parsons and Prigatano 1978). While

Table 7.1 Demographic and Neurological Characteristics of NRP Patients

Patient	Age[a]	Sex	Years of Education	Occupation at Time of Injury	Chronicity[b]	Length of Coma[c] (Retrospective)	Posttrauma Seizure Disorder	Residual Paresis	Residual Aphasia and/or Dysarthria	Clinical Diagnosis[d]
1	32	M	18	Vocational rehabilitation counselor	22	>3 days <7 days	No	No	No	SCC[d]
2	18	M	12	College student	6	>7 days <14 days	Yes	No	No	SCC&BSC[e]
3	21	M	12	Machinist	10	>7 days	Yes	Yes	Yes	SCC
4	37	F	14	Housewife	18	>21 days	No	Yes	No	SCC&BSC
5	37	M	14	Technical salesman	8	>24 hrs <3 days	No	Yes	No	SCC
6	20	M	11	High school student	36	>21 days	No	Yes	Yes	SCC&BSC
7	19	M	12	Oilfield worker	12	>3 days <7 days	No	Yes	No	SCC&BSC
8	19	M	12	High school student	10	>24 hrs <3 days	Yes	Yes	Yes	SCC
9	20	M	12	Machinist	6	>3 days <7 days	No	Yes	No	SCC
10	22	F	13	Sales clerk	54	>24 hrs <3 days	No	No	No	SCC
11	25	M	14	Self-employed businessman	54	"several weeks"	No	No	No	SCC
12	20	M	12	Oilfield worker	15	>24 hrs <3 days	No	No	No	SCC
13	21	F	12	Custodian	9	>24 hrs <3 days	No	Yes	No	SCC
14	34	M	18	Personnel director	13	>14days <21 days	No	No	No	SCC
15	19	M	12	Army private	14	"several weeks"	No	Yes	Yes	SCC&BSC
16	44	M	12	Mechanical engineer	7	>7days <14 days	No	Yes	Yes	BSC
17	37	M	14	Cattleman	13	>24 hrs <3 days	No	Yes	No	SCC
18	24	M	12	High school student	81	"several weeks"	No	Yes	Yes	SCC&BSC
Mean	26.1		12.5		21.6					
SD	8.3		3.3		21.0					

[a] Age at time of entering NRP.
[b] Time since injury, in months.
[c] Retrospective analysis of medical charts.
[d] Severe cerebral contusion.
[e] Brain-stem contusion.

121

every attempt was made to select controls blind to their general outcome status, in some cases this was impossible, given the authors' familiarity with certain individuals. Recommendation to participate in the NRP program was made to many of these seventeen controls following initial neuropsychological examination, but for a variety of reasons these recommendations were not followed. In general, the controls were similar to the NRP patients in that they had suffered serious head injuries and were having difficulties adjusting to their residual deficits. Five had a posttraumatic seizure disorder, five had residual paresis, and six had residual signs of aphasia and/or dysarthria. Therefore, the groups were relatively matched on gross neurological sequelae. (See Table 7.2).

Neuropsychological Tests

NRP patients received a comprehensive neuropsychological examination prior to their entering the program. A repeat examination took place upon completion of six months of rehabilitation. Control subjects received the same basic battery of neuropsychological tests, although the assessments were not always as complete and the intertest interval was more variable than that of the NRP subjects. From the core neuropsychological test battery, the following measures were extracted for analysis in the present study:

1. The Verbal IQ, Performance IQ, Vocabulary, Block Design, and Digit Symbol subtests of the Wechsler Adult Intelligence Scale or WAIS-R (Wechsler 1955, 1981).
2. The Memory Quotient, Logical Memory, and Visual Reproduction subtests of the Wechsler Memory Scale (Wechsler 1945). In addition, the number of difficult paired associates learned over the three trials of the Association Learning subtest of the Wechsler Memory Scale was calculated (Prigatano 1978).
3. The Trail Making Test, Finger Tapping Test and Tactual Performance Test of the Halstead-Reitan Neuropsychological Test Battery (Reitan and Davison 1974).
4. The Russell-Neuringer Average Impairment Rating (AIR), based on the extended Halstead-Reitan Battery (Russell et al. 1970), when sufficient test data were present, to serve as a global index of overall neuropsychological status.

Personality Tests

Assessment of personality characteristics of the NRP patients was undertaken with the Katz-R Adjustment Scale Relatives' Form. This standardized instrument provides a means by which significant others can rate the personality and social behavior of the patients (Fordyce et al. 1983). Scores

Table 7.2 Demographic and Neurological Characteristics of Control Subjects

Patient	Age[a]	Sex	Years of Education	Occupation at Time of Injury	Chronicity[b]	Length of Coma[c] (Retrospective)	Posttrauma Seizure Disorder	Residual Paresis	Residual Aphasia and/or Dysarthria	Clinical Diagnosis
1	23	M	14	College student	7	>24 hrs <3 days	Yes	No	Yes	SCC[d]
2	26	M	12	Construction worker	12	Unknown	No	No	No	SCC
3	16	F	11	High school student	12	>3 days <7 days	No	No	No	SCC
4	22	M	10	Navy recruit	13	>7 days <14 days	Yes	Yes	Yes	SCC
5	28	M	16	Counselor for juvenile delinquents	9	>7 days <14 days	No	No	Mild anomia	SCC
6	25	M	12	Salesman for oilfield equipment	8	>24 hrs	No	Mild right hand weakness	No	SCC
7	36	M	0	Oilfield worker	8	>24 hrs <3 days	No	No	No	SCC
8	23	M	11	Plumber	12	>7 days <14 days	Yes	Yes	Yes	SCC&BSC[e]
9	24	M	12	Oilfield worker	18	>7 days <14 days	No	No	No	SCC&BSC
10	20	M	14	College student	5	>24 hrs	Yes	No	No	SCC
11	15	F	9	High school student	5	>2 wks	No	No	No	SCC
12	21	M	11	Army private	8	Unknown	No	Yes	No	SCC
13	22	M	14	College student	11	>2 wks	No	Yes	Yes	SCC&BSC
14	25	M	12	Pipe fitter	8	Unknown	Yes	No	No	SCC
15	23	M	11	Oil company serviceman	25	>7 days <14 days	No	No	Yes	SCC&BSC
16	19	M	12	High school student	20	>7 days <14 days	No	Yes	No	SCC
17	26	M	15	Farmer	44	>24 hrs <3 days	No	No	No	SCC&BSC
Mean	23.5		11.5		15.9					
SD	5.1		3.5		13.6					

[a] Age at first examination.
[b] Time since injury, in months.
[c] Retrospective analysis of medical charts.
[d] Severe cerebral contusion.
[e] Brain-stem contusion.

were converted to age-corrected Z scores on the basis of the normative population (Hogarty and Katz 1971). Unfortunately, Katz data were not available for all control patients.

The Follow-up Interview

NRP and control patients were contacted by telephone during the months of April and May 1983. Each patient and, when possible, a relative were interviewed using a structured interview form developed by the NRP staff. Responses to questions concerning current work status and the work history, since the time of the last examination, were extracted for the present evaluation. If there were questions concerning the reliability of the patient's narrative, a vigorous attempt was made to obtain the same information from a relative.

Analysis and Findings of the Neuropsychological Tests

While every attempt was made to match control subjects on what was felt to be important nontreatment variables affecting outcome from brain injury, it proved nearly impossible to do this adequately. As a result, post hoc statistical measures were undertaken to reduce the potential influence of confounding variables. This was accomplished through analysis of covariance, with the pool of covariates including age, educational level, time since injury of the first evaluation (chronicity), and time between the first and second evaluations (intertest interval). To control for differences in initial level of impairment, the pretest performance for each neuropsychological measure also served as a covariate. Analyses were completed only on the posttest scores, after adjusting for the various covariates. This procedure helped control for changes in test performance directly related to initial levels of impairment (Green 1978) and allowed for generally greater statistical precision relative to the more traditional methods of analyzing change scores. Statistical analyses of each neuropsychological variable were completed only for those subjects who had both pretest and posttest score values.

The general analysis of covariance procedure was as follows: First, a stepwise regression procedure (Barr et al. 1976) was employed to isolate the covariates significantly related to each individual posttest neuropsychological score. The grouping factor (NRP versus control) and initial pretest score values were "forced" into the regression model. After these sources of variance were entered, the remaining covariates (age, education, chronicity, intertest interval) and their interactions were analyzed to isolate which contributed additional independent variance to the regression model given the previously entered covariates. The covariate generating the largest F statistic for variance added was entered into the model first. This process was repeated until the remaining covariates and their interactions could not generate a significant "F statistic to enter the model" of 0.3 or less. Thus, for each neuropsychological posttest measure, a unique group of variables was identified, which covaried with the particular measure independent of the major grouping factor (NRP versus control).

Second, analyses of covariance were subsequently completed on each neuropsychological test measure. As indicated, pretest scores were always employed as the first covariate in the model. Subsequently, the additional covariates and/or their interactions identified in the preceding stepwise regression analysis were also entered into the analyses of covariance model. The complete model for each variable then yielded a comparison of posttest neuropsychological scores between NRP and control patients adjusted for initial test performance and any other uncontrolled source of variance identified.

On the basis of the follow-up interview, the NRP patients were dichotomized into two groups, based on their employment histories since discharge from the program. The employed group consisted of patients that remained productive for 75 percent or more of the time since discharge. The unemployed group were those patients who failed to maintain productive activities for 75 percent of the time following discharge. Neuropsychological test and personality measures were then reassessed for these two groups to determine whether these variables could discriminate the work outcome groups. Analyses of covariance were performed on posttest scores for the neuropsychological and personality measures (after adjusting for pretest levels).

With a few exceptions, the control patients were similar to the NRP patients on the matching variables. NRP patients were, on the average, 26.1 years old ($SD = 8.3$) compared with 23.5 ($SD = 5.1$) for controls. The two groups were also similar with respect to the years of education attained. The NRP subjects averaged 12.5 years of school ($SD = 3.3$), the controls averaged 11.5 years ($SD = 3.5$). The two groups were similar in sex composition, with fifteen males and three females comprising the NRP subject population and fifteen males and two females comprising the control population. The slight differences between groups in age, education, and sex composition were not statistically significant (i.e., $p < .05$).

There was a tendency for the NRP subjects to be more chronic than controls. At first testing, they averaged 21.6 months since injury ($SD = 21$), compared with 15.9 months ($SD = 13.6$) for controls. This difference fell short of statistical significance because of the sample size. The intertest interval did reliably discriminate the two groups, however ($F = 3.98$, $DF = 1/33$, $p = .05$). NRP patients, on the average, had less time between testings (7.5 months), compared with controls (12.6 months). The shorter initial chronicities and the longer intertest intervals would tend to favor

Table 7.3 Average Wechsler Test Scores of NRP Patients and Control Subjects before and after Treatment

Test	NRP (N)	Before	After	Controls (N)	Before	After
WAIS[a]						
VIQ[b]	(16)	97.2	100.4	(12)	98.3	102.3
PIQ[b]	(17)	86.8	95.5	(14)	85.8	90.6
Vocabulary[c]	(15)	9.0	9.8	(10)	9.6	9.2
Block Design[c]	(18)	8.9	10.9	(15)	8.0	9.4
Digit Symbol[c]	(18)	6.3	7.5	(15)	6.3	6.7
WMS[d]						
WMQ	(18)	85.4	94.9	(13)	90.8	92.8
Logical Memory[e]	(18)	6.9	8.0	(13)	7.0	6.8
Visual Reproduction[e]	(18)	4.3	5.6	(13)	6.4	6.2
No. hard associates[f]	(18)	7.6	10.1	(13)	7.9	9.3

[a] Both WAIS and WAIS-R versions were employed.
[b] Prorated IQ values based on 5/6 verbal and 4/5 performance subtests.
[c] Scale scores.
[d] Wechsler Memory Scale.
[e] Raw scores.
[f] Total number of four hard associates learned over three trials.

relatively greater spontaneous neuropsychological recovery among the controls relative to the NRP patients (Bond and Brooks 1976). In any event, these two variables were utilized as covariates in various statistical analyses, particularly for test scores for neuropsychological measures.

There was a trend for rehabilitation patients to be more neuropsychologically impaired than controls. The NRP patients obtained an initial mean Average Impairment Rating of 2.35 ($N = 17$). For those control subjects for whom an AIR could be calculated ($N = 10$), the AIR was somewhat lower (AIR = 1.82). While this difference did not reach statistical significance, the initial level of impairment was deemed an important control variable and employed as a covariate in various analyses.

The NRP patients showed a trend for better neuropsychological functioning at posttest, compared with controls. These improvements were obtained after adjusting for the effects of initial level of performance and, where appropriate, age, education, chronicity, and test interval. Tables 7.3 and 7.4 present mean values for the two groups, pretest and posttest. The analyses of covariance indicated significantly better posttest performance for NRP subjects relative to controls for the following neuropsychological variables: WAIS Performance IQ ($F = 9.74$, $DF = 1/21$, $p = .005$), WAIS Block Design Scale Score ($F = 22.81$, $DF = 1/26$, $p = .0001$), and Wechsler Memory Quotient ($F = 5.27$, $DF = 1/27$, $p = .03$). In addition, there were nearly significant trends for NRP subjects to be less impaired at posttest,

Table 7.4 Average Neuropsychological Test Scores of NRP Patients and Control Subjects before and after Treatment (Selected Halstead-Reitan Tests)

	NRP			Controls		
Test	(N)	Before	After	(N)	Before	After
AIR[a]	(17)	2.35	2.09	(9)	1.98	1.77
Tapping[b]						
DH[c]	(16)	42.60	44.20	(9)	36.20	36.80
NDH[d]	(16)	39.00	42.20	(9)	36.80	38.30
TPT[e]						
DH[c]	(12)	462.40	485.10	(6)	410.30	403.50
NDH[d]	(12)	447.90	385.90	(6)	386.50	385.70
Trail Making[f]						
Part A	(18)	60.80	45.30	(11)	49.30	44.30
Part B	(17)	163.20	133.20	(11)	125.80	110.40

[a] Russell-Neuringer Average Impairment Rating.
[b] Finger Tapping Test, number of finger taps in ten seconds.
[c] Dominant hand.
[d] Nondominant hand.
[e] Tactual Performance Test, time to complete tactile form board in seconds. Dominant hand on first trial, nondominant hand on second trial (600 second limit per trial).
[f] Trail Making Test, time in seconds.

compared with controls, on the WAIS Digit Symbol subtest ($F = 3.48$, $DF = 1/25$, $p = .07$), the Tactual Performance Test time for the nondominant hand ($F = 4.73$, $DF = 1/9$, $p = .06$), and the Russell-Neuringer Average Impairment Rating ($F = 3.85$, $DF = 1/21$, $p = .06$). Only for the time to complete the Tactual Performance Test with the dominant hand did controls perform better than NRP subjects ($F = 6.84$, $DF = 1/9$, $p = .03$). None of the remaining analyses of covariance identified significant posttest performance differences between the two groups of subjects. Figure 7.1 presents pretest-posttest change scores on certain neuropsychological variables for NRP patients and controls.

Personality Test Findings

NRP patients showed more improvement in personality functioning, compared with controls. Reports by their relatives indicated lower ratings (by at least one Z score) on helplessness, degree of social withdrawal, signs of general psychopathology, and restlessness or hyperactivity. Mean age-corrected Z score values for both groups of patients are presented in Table 7.5. NRP patients and controls were also compared as to whether they simply showed increases or decreases on each of the thirteen Katz-R Adjustment Scales. The chi-square analysis, using the Yates Correction, approached significance ($X^2 = 3.46$, $p = .06$). NRP patients showed declines on twelve of the thirteen dimensions and increases in only two dimensions, one of which reflects improvement in stability. In contrast, controls

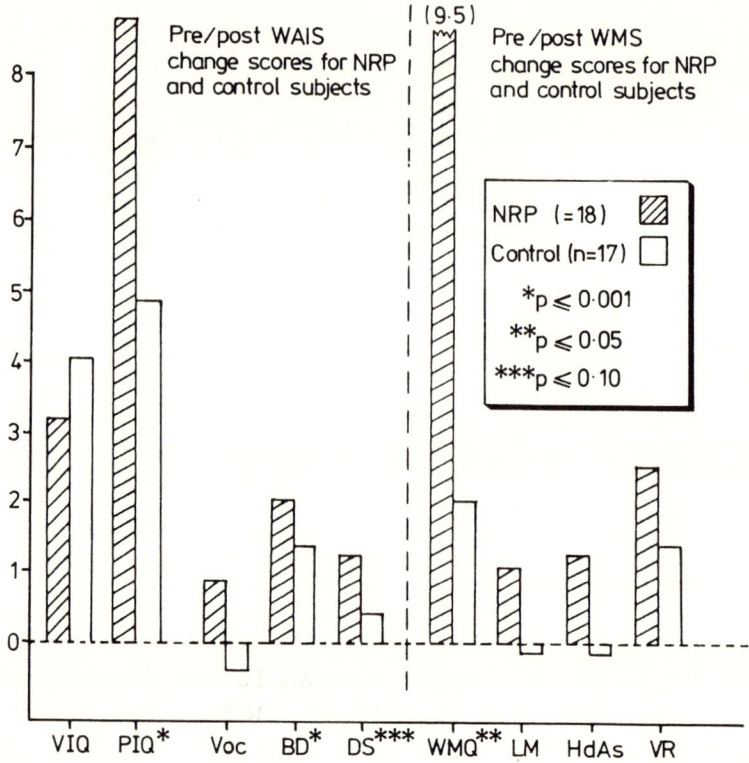

Figure 7.1. Scores on Intelligence and Memory Tests of NRP Patients and Control Subjects. VIQ = Verbal Intelligence Quotient; PIQ = Performance Intelligence Quotient; Voc = Vocabulary; BD = Block Design; DS = Digit Symbol; WMQ = Wechsler Memory Quotient; LM = Logical Memory; HdAs = Hard Associates; VR = Visual Reproduction.

showed declines on eight dimensions and increases on six dimensions, only one of which reflects improvement.

Work Status during Follow-up

NRP patients and controls were compared on whether they were gainfully employed (part-time or full-time) or actively engaged in a realistic school program at the time of follow-up. Nine of the eighteen NRP patients (50 percent) were classified as productive on this basis, nine were not. Five of the controls (36 percent) were productive at follow-up, eight were not. Three were lost to follow-up.

The neuropsychological and personality characteristics of the nine NRP patients who were working at the time of follow-up were contrasted to those NRP patients who had failed to be gainfully employed. There were no significant differences in educational level, age, or chronicity for the patients who were employed during follow-up, compared with those who

Table 7.5 Katz-R Adjustment Scale Z Scores (Relatives' Ratings of Psychosocial Adjustment) of NRP Patients and Control Subjects before and after Treatment

Subtest	NRP ($N=13$)			Controls ($N=6$)		
	Before	After	Change	Before	After	Change
Belligerence	1.44	0.58	−0.86	2.86	2.26	−0.40
Verbal expansiveness	1.15	0.99	−0.16	3.01	3.04	+0.03
Negativism	2.18	1.20	−0.98	2.96	3.31	+0.35
Helplessness	2.42	1.13	−1.29	3.43	2.47	−0.96
Suspiciousness	1.91	2.66	+0.75	2.47	2.67	+0.20
Anxiety	0.67	0.54	−0.13	1.25	0.24	−1.01
Withdrawal/retardation	3.67	2.13	−1.54	3.17	3.26	+0.09
General psychopathology	5.87	4.38	−1.49	8.14	6.41	−1.73
Nervousness	2.15	0.94	−1.21	0.36	1.31	+0.95
Confusion	2.02	1.03	−0.99	4.86	1.04	−3.82
Bizarreness	0.47	0.01	−0.48	1.46	1.29	−0.17
Hyperactivity	1.94	0.79	−1.15	3.58	2.29	−1.29
Stability	−3.89	−2.98	+0.91	−4.06	−3.89	+0.17

Note: Scores are mean age-corrected scores.

were not employed. Similarly, while there was a trend on some measures for the unemployed group to be more impaired in neuropsychological functioning, there were no statistically significant differences between the two groups on any of the neuropsychological measures. In contrast, relatives' ratings of emotional and motivational functioning, on the Katz-R Adjustment Scale, did discriminate the two outcome groups. There was a tendency for the unemployed group to be rated as more deviant at *pretest* on most of the clinical dimensions of the Katz-R. Only for the stability measure was the difference statistically significant ($F=5.17$, $DF=1/16$, $p=.04$). At posttest, however, there were much greater differences. The unemployed group was rated as more deviant on most of the clinical dimensions, compared with the employed group. Statistically significant differences were obtained for the verbal expansiveness measure ($F=4.93$, $DF=1/11$, $p=.05$), the negativism scale ($F=5.67$, $DF=1/11$, $p=.04$), the general psychopathology measure ($F=15.9$, $DF=1/11$, $p=.0003$), the hyperactivity measure ($F=31.64$, $DF=1/11$, $p=.0002$), and the stability measure ($F=47.41$, $DF=1/11$, $p=.0001$).

Analyses of covariance completed on posttest scores after adjusting for initial test levels revealed some interesting differences between groups. Employed patients show *greater improvement* on most of the neuropsychological tests. Significant differences between the two groups, however, were obtained only for the WAIS Digit Symbol subtest ($F=10.39$, $DF=1/15$, $p=.0006$), the Wechsler Memory Quotient ($F=6.04$, $DF=1/15$, $p=.03$), the Visual Reproduction subtest of the Wechsler Memory Scale ($F=4.56$, $DF=1/15$, $p=.05$), and the number of difficult paired associates learned from the Associate Learning subtest ($F=7.73$,

$DF = 1/15$, $p = .01$). For the Katz Adjustment Scale measures, following adjustment for initial values, the employed NRP patients tended to show greater improvement on the general psychopathology scale ($F = 16.44$, $DF = 1/10$, $p = .0002$), the hyperactivity scale ($F = 29.16$, $DF = 1/10$, $p = .0003$), and the stability scale ($F = 40.51$, $DF = 1/10$, $p = .0001$), compared with the unemployed NRP patients.

The Effectiveness of Neuropsychological Rehabilitation

These preliminary findings on the effectiveness of an intensive neuropsychological rehabilitation program for chronic and moderately to severely impaired closed-head-injury patients suggest that such training may improve neuropsychological status and reduce emotional distress. Of course, these findings need to be replicated in other settings, as well as obtained in a larger sample of patients. The data are encouraging because they document modest but statistically reliable improvements on standardized neuropsychological tests. Past the period of so-called spontaneous recovery, cognitive retraining activities appear to help patients improve their speed of information-processing (as reflected particularly by the Performance IQ score). Improved neuropsychological status was also related to eventual gainful employment. The data further suggest that memory skills are very important in this regard. Clinically, it appears that NRP patients are more organized and less confused, and this may lead to better test performance. It will be important to assess longitudinally whether these improvements continue to maintain themselves or whether periodic retraining activities are needed to sustain them.

These data, and clinical observations, also suggest that substantial improvement in interpersonal skills and reduction of emotional distress are possible with this type of intervention. Patients can be helped to be less helpless, less socially withdrawn, and less hyperactive. They also can be taught to be more reliable and less anxious and depressed. These improvements appear to be related to reducing cognitive confusion and teaching patients to compensate for neuropsychological impairments. Teaching patients to recognize their own form of the catastrophic reaction (Prigatano, in press) appears to be important in enhancing their social adaptation. Without such therapeutic intervention, emotional disturbances do not get better on their own (Fordyce et al. 1983). It appears, therefore, that one of the most important benefits of the intensive NRP is improvement of psychosocial adjustment.

Both the neuropsychological and personality findings reaffirm what has been previously reported. Closed-head-injury patients who can learn information with practice and demonstrate reduced memory deficits and personality difficulties generally have a better work adjustment (Bond 1975;

Weddell et al. 1980; Bruckner and Randle 1972). It is especially interesting, from a neuropsychological testing point of view, that improvement on the WAIS Digit Symbol subtest score may be a powerful discriminator between those closed-head-injury patients who return to work and those who do not. This test measures, among other things, the ability to learn with practice and the speed of new learning. It does not sample higher abstract reasoning or problem-solving skills. If the patient is within the lower limits of normal on this test by the end of rehabilitation, it suggests that the patient has the basic cognitive capacities to be taught work skills and to be competitive, in terms of efficiency of functioning (at least for some jobs). These data would seem to relate well to other research relating Performance IQ to vocational adjustment (Heaton and Pendleton 1981).

While the above findings are encouraging, the work outcome statistics on sustained employment are sobering. Initially, it was our impression that between 60 and 65 percent of the patients would work or were working shortly after their neuropsychological rehabilitation program ended. With the passage of time, however, that percentage dropped to 50 percent. Moreover, 36 percent of the controls return to gainful employment without intensive rehabilitation. This figure is compatible with other reports of between 33 and 40 percent gainful employment with traditional rehabilitative care. Why is there only a 14 percent difference in treated versus nontreated patients in terms of work status, and can this figure be improved?

The methods used in our closed-head-injury program were primarily designed to enhance neuropsychological function (particularly speed of information-processing) and personality adjustment. To some degree, these goals were accomplished. It was hoped, however, that this would automatically lead to greater work productivity. We now see this as a somewhat naive assumption. Improving neuropsychological status and personality skills is necessary, but not sufficient for accomplishing a productive life-style. Specific training in this area is needed if the desired goal is to get the patient back to work and to keep him or her gainfully employed. The NRP has been redesigned to include a work trial and teaching of job maintenance skills (see Chapter 8 and Appendix C). With this addition, we are hoping to achieve a greater percentage of sustained independent living and productivity in our patients.

Patients who seem to have benefited most from the NRP generally have the following test characteristics. The Average Impairment Rating is usually no greater than 2.00 to 2.25 at the onset of the rehabilitation program. This is usually about twelve to eighteen months after traumatic head injury. The Digit Symbol subtest score is usually at least 6 at the beginning of the rehabilitation program (it moves to 8 or greater by the end of the program). Rote verbal learning, as measured by the Associate Learning subtest of the Wechsler Memory Scale, approaches normal limits. Performance IQ typically is at least in the 80s.

From the perspective of personality functioning, employable patients typically have affective disturbance, which represents problems in coping (e.g., the catastrophic reaction). Their problems with anxiety, anger, depression, and so on, are in response to not knowing how to handle the cognitive, perceptual, and motor limitations imposed by their brain injury. Preexisting significant characterological and/or personality disturbances foster a poor outcome.

A good work history prior to the traumatic head injury, and a supportive social milieu outside the program (which encourages the patient to take realistic steps in returning to work), are also vital. In this regard, it is not necessary that the patient have a great deal of formal education. It is more important that the patient have a stable work history. Patients who have a sporadic work history usually have poor treatment outcome.

Finally, the patients who seem to have neurologically based problems in awareness and who can be helped to become aware of and to accept residual neuropsychological deficits make the best candidates for this type of program. Typically, these individuals show a willingness to use compensatory methods to get around deficits that have an impact on their home life and work life. The problems of awareness and acceptance are crucial concerns that need constant rehabilitative attention.

Some patients, who initially appeared to be ideal candidates for this type of neuropsychological rehabilitation program, failed. Others, who looked as if they were going to be poor candidates, succeeded. The defining characteristics of those patients who would benefit from this type of program are only broadly known. A successful outcome appears to be the result of a combination of factors, including the type and severity of brain injury, the premorbid characteristics of the patients, the skill and dedication of therapists, and the local social and economic conditions that determine whether gainful employment is a practical goal. We are encouraged with these initial findings, insofar as they suggest that improvement can take place past the period of spontaneous recovery for many brain-injured patients. Also, with the necessary training, the rate of gainful employment may be substantially better than what has been previously thought.

Summary

Cognitive and personality disturbances following severe closed head injury in young adults are clearly associated with poor rehabilitation outcome. Yet systematic programs for dealing with these disturbances have generally not appeared. The present chapter briefly described the initial outcome data on eighteen closed-head-injury patients in the Neuropsychological

Rehabilitation Program at Presbyterian Hospital and seventeen untreated controls. Greater improvement in neuropsychological functioning occurred in the NRP patient group on selected variables, but generally the effects were modest. However, emotional distress substantially decreased in treated patients. Some 50 percent of the NRP patients maintained productivity 75 percent of the time or more following rehabilitation, compared with 36 percent of the controls. Treatment successes showed fewer personality disturbances than treatment failures, and better learning and memory scores posttreatment.

CHAPTER **8**
Modification of the Neuropsychological Rehabilitation Program at Presbyterian Hospital, Oklahoma City

George P. Prigatano

The Modified Program

Since the initial papers on which the preceding chapters are based were written, changes in our approach to working with brain-injured patients have occurred. While the intensive, integrated-treatment approach is still seen as a necessary component to successful rehabilitation, it is not sufficient by itself. What Goldstein (1942) recognized years ago we and others are starting to reaffirm. Brain-injured patients need a guided and at times protected work trial if the ultimate goal is for them to return to the community as productive individuals.

This is not an easy task. Besides the logistics of identifying appropriate job settings, conducting a job analysis, and comparing a given job's requirements with a given patient's competencies, the community as a whole must be able to take these individuals back into its midst. This involves both economic and political issues. We are working with a business advisory committee and administrators at Presbyterian Hospital to make this transition possible. Appendix C presents a description of our revised Neuropsychological Rehabilitation Program. The program now consists of working with patients primarily in cognitive retraining and psychotherapy for four hours a day. The afternoons are reserved for actual work trials. Initially, patients are placed in voluntary positions; it is hoped that they will move into paid, part-time employment. This gives us an opportunity to take actual work behaviors that are both adaptive and nonadaptive and deal with them within the context of the Neuropsychological Rehabilitation Program. This information can be used to help patients see practically what they need to do in order to improve work behaviors and be able not only to obtain a job but to maintain one as well. This change in the NRP followed the outcome data compiled in 1984 (see Chapter 7), which convinced us of the importance of a work trial.

The description of the present program presented in Appendix C demonstrates the type of information that needs to be communicated to patients, families, referral sources, and third-party payors regarding the intentions of a neuropsychological rehabilitation oriented program. The material in Appendix C is also provided because it conveys the transition that our program has undergone and therefore might be useful to other therapists in the field.

Clinical Observations

We have also learned some important lessons regarding the treatment team. Each therapist has his or her own personal reaction to this type of intensive work. If the staff take their clinical obligations seriously, they eventually experience problems that mirror or reflect what the families of patients go through. There is often an initial excitement over trying something new, which eventually gives way to the monotony of dealing with brain-dysfunctional patients. Also, the staff can feel embarrassed, angry, and hopeless. Patients' inappropriate social comments, both in the treatment setting and outside it, can have a wearing effect on both family and staff. Even if one understands the causes of these behavioral problems, the problems have their effect on staff and family.

The staff need to recognize these reactions and establish a reasonable work commitment to the patient and family in order to have the rehabilitation progress at a reasonable rate. This requires that the staff be realistic in their assessment of what they can offer patients and enter into a fair and honest contractual arrangement with them.

If the staff make reasonable commitments and are given the necessary support from their co-workers as well as from hospital administrators, they can embrace this work with enthusiasm, energy, and creativity. Just like family members, however, they need a break from the demands of this type of work, and this must be built into their work schedules. Bond (1983) and Gans (1983) elegantly describe the difficulties that families and staff experience in working with brain-dysfunctional patients.

The challenge of the future is to consider the needs of patients, family members, and staff in a manner that allows for the development of the most effective and yet cost-efficient treatment interventions. A system of accepting brain-injured patients back into the community is vital, not only for patients but also for society at large.

Final comments center on the clinical impressions concerning the determinants of neuropsychological rehabilitation outcome. From February 1980 to February 1984, some 44 patients entered the NRP. Four of these patients dropped out, three of those during the first year of operation. In each case the dropout had become very disturbed with the feedback that he

Table 8.1 Demographic and Neurological Characteristics of 40 Patients Completing the NRP (February 1980 to February 1984)

Item	Successes ($N=11$)		Intermediates ($N=12$)		Failures ($N=17$)	
	Mean	SD	Mean	SD	Mean	SD
Age	26.6	8.6	25.6	6.9	28.1	7.4
Education	13.4	2.5	13.0	4.0	12.8	2.1
Chronicity[a]	39.4	37.4	20.4	18.6	40.6	74.8
Sex	M = 82%		M = 75%		M = 82%	
	F = 18%		F = 25%		F = 18%	
Diagnosis						
Severe craniocerebral trauma	9		8		12	
Ruptured aneurysm	2		2		1	
Tumor	0		1		2	
Other	0		1		1	
Ruptured AVM[b]	0		0		1	

[a] Months since time of injury and entry into NRP.
[b] Arteriovenous malformation.

or she was receiving regarding the difficulties secondary to brain injury. One of the first four has been lost to follow-up, but the remaining three continue to have major adjustment problems. In retrospect, all four had significant pretrauma interpersonal adjustment difficulties.

Of the forty patients who stayed in the intensive NRP, the treatment staff considered eleven to be clear successes (28 percent) and seventeen to be clear treatment failures (42 percent). The remaining twelve (or 30 percent) were considered to show some benefit from treatment but were in between any clear classification of success versus failure. They were designated "intermediates."

Classification of patients as "successes," "failures," or "intermediates" was made by the staff collectively. The degree of independence, ability to become productive, understanding and acceptance of residual strengths and limitations, and reasonable interpersonal judgment were the guiding considerations. The staff who classified patients consisted of three clinical neuropsychologists and one research psychologist, one speech and language pathologist, and one occupational therapist.

Table 8.1 lists the demographic and neurological characteristics of these patients. No significant age, education, or sex difference existed between the groups, but treatment successes and failures were clearly more chronic. However, there was great variability between subjects in each classification concerning time since injury, so this is a tentative conclusion.

Some 27 percent (three out of eleven) of the successes had residual hemi-

Table 8.2 Mean Neuropsychological Test Scores of NRP Patients

Test	First Exam (at entry)		Second Exam (at completion)	
	Successes	Failures	Successes	Failures
Wechsler Tests				
Verbal IQ	100.70	91.10	104.20	95.90
Performance IQ	89.00	80.60	99.20	87.20
Vocabulary subtest	10.00	9.20	10.10	9.50
Block Design subtest	9.60	7.70	12.10	8.30
Digit Symbol subtest	6.20	5.20	8.10	6.10
Memory Quotient	85.80	82.60	97.60	89.60
Logical Memory	5.60	7.30	7.60	7.70
No. hard associates	4.00	3.10	5.80	3.60
Visual Reproduction	7.80	6.70	11.00	8.80
Halstead-Reitan Tests				
Trails Part A	59.70	61.90	40.60	56.20
Trails Part B	167.80	155.50	128.10	158.10
Category Test	46.00	62.00	43.00	56.80
Tactual Performance (right)	422.30	562.60	486.90	534.63
Tactual Performance (left)	436.50	534.50	386.40	498.27
Finger Tapping (right)	41.50	38.70	40.80	40.20
Finger Tapping (left)	40.20	34.80	42.10	35.10
AIR	2.12	2.75	1.94	2.56

paresis or hemiplegia. Some 17 percent (two out of twelve) and 29 percent (five out of seventeen) of the intermediates and failures, respectively, had similar residual motor difficulties. Two out of the eleven successes (18 percent) had residual language difficulties, compared with 0 percent in the other two groups. Thus, the capacity to "walk and talk" was not a significant predictor of the ability to benefit from the NRP.

Generally, the successes had less neuropsychological impairment than the failures. The intermediates fell in between these two groups. On all but one of the seventeen neuropsychological measures used, successes had better scores (i.e., less impairment) than failures at the beginning of the NRP (see Table 8.2). By the completion of the program, the same pattern held.

Three-by-two analyses of variance (i.e., successes vs. intermediates vs. failures × exam 1 vs. exam 2) generally failed to produce statistically significant findings. This was because of the large variability in test scores for patients in each group as well as the relatively small Ns. However, some interesting findings emerged. As would be expected from the data in Table 8.2, an effect was frequently observed between the first and second testings. This may be solely the result of the effect of practice, or it may reflect some modest improvement in neuropsychological status over time and treatment in our patient group.

Measures that showed a trend among the three groups were the WAIS

Table 8.3 Mean Katz-R Test Scores of NRP Patients

Subtest	First Exam		Second Exam	
	Successes ($N=11$)	Failures ($N=14$)	Successes ($N=7$)	Failures ($N=10$)
Belligerence	0.59	2.05	−0.30	1.77
Verbal expansiveness	0.46	1.18	−0.33	2.45
Negativism	0.26	2.17	−0.14	1.83
Helplessness	2.39	2.54	1.09	2.97
Suspiciousness	1.18	2.50	1.45	2.77
Anxiety	1.13	1.50	0.72	0.94
Withdrawal	2.93	4.04	3.23	3.45
General psychopathology	5.03	6.65	2.73	7.44
Nervousness	2.33	1.75	0.83	1.87
Confusion	1.85	1.99	1.54	2.51
Bizarreness	0.31	0.66	0.05	0.13
Hyperactivity	1.13	1.41	0.18	1.61
Stability	−2.13	−5.09	−2.50	−5.05

Note: Scores are age-corrected Z scores. Any Z value of 1.96 is significant at the 0.5 level, compared with age-matched normals using Hogarty and Katz (1971) norms.

Block Design subtest ($F = 2.87$, $p = .06$), the number of hard paired-associates learned on the Wechsler Memory Scale ($F = 2.24$, $p = .12$), and the WAIS Performance IQ ($F = 2.15$, $p = .13$). These measures generally reflect basic memory skills, ability to perform under time pressure, and visual constructive abilities. It has been our clinical impression that these are key elements to neuropsychological rehabilitation success. Table 8.2 illustrates, for example, that as a group the Digit Symbol subtest score improved by two scale scores for the successes and was in the low-average range by the completion of the NRP. In contrast, as a group, failures only improved by one scale score and the mean value was notably below average. As Chapter 7 indicated, significant improvement on the WAIS Digit Symbol subtest scores was clearly related to vocational success in the first group of head-injured patients systematically studied. The same was found for some memory scores and personality variables.

The neuropsychological test findings make it clear that while the degree of neuropsychological impairment is an important determinant of the treatment outcome, other variables may be equally important. Moreover, the relative strengths of different predictors of treatment outcome may be different for failures and successes. The case material of the seventeen treatment failures was collectively and simultaneously reviewed by the NRP staff. In order of importance, the factors that seemed to be associated with treatment failures were:

1. "Significant" cognitive disturbance, which reflected memory deficit,

Table 8.4 Duncan Multiple-range Scores on Katz-R Data for NRP Patients

Subtests	Successes	Intermediates	Failures
Belligerence	0.48 (A)[a]	0.65 (A)	1.93 (A)
Verbal expansiveness	0.15 (A)	0.63 (A) (B)	1.71 (B)
Negativism	0.10 (A)	1.91 (B)	2.03 (B)
Helplessness	1.89 (A)	2.52 (A)	2.72 (A)
Suspiciousness	1.28 (A)	1.89 (A)	2.61 (A)
Anxiety	0.97 (A)	0.77 (A)	1.29 (A)
Withdrawal	3.05 (A)	3.79 (A)	3.79 (A)
General psychopathology	4.14 (A)	5.21 (A) (B)	6.98 (B)
Nervousness	0.64 (A)	1.75 (A)	1.82 (A)
Confusion	1.73 (A)	1.92 (A)	2.21 (A)
Bizarreness	0.21 (A)	0.44 (A)	0.63 (A)
Hyperactivity	0.76 (A)	1.44 (A)	1.49 (A)
Stability	−2.43 (A)	−3.25 (A) (B)	−5.07 (B)

Note: Scores are age-corrected Z-scores.

[a] Letters that are the same reflect no significant difference ($p \geq .05$). Letters that are different do reflect statistical significance ($p \leq .05$).

disorders of judgment, impulsivity, poor organization and planning, and nonaphasic communication difficulties
2. Inadequate postinjury coping mechanisms, which included major difficulties in becoming aware of the residual deficits, and an inability to accept and develop methods of compensation
3. Clinical evidence of premorbid characterological disturbances, which contributed to poor *premorbid* job stability, interpersonal relationships, and legal entanglements
4. Significant sensory-motor disturbances, which precluded ambulation and/or effective use of the upper extremities

These factors impressed us as key elements of predicting treatment failure. In contrast, as clinicians, we have been impressed with the role of "social competency" in determining treatment success. While certainly a few of the treatment successes had "significant" or "severe" cognitive disturbances and a few had poor premorbid adjustment difficulties, each of the successes found a way of coping with his or her deficits. Moreover, the coping strategies were acceptable to the treatment staff and others. Thus, the patient did not alienate others, despite the expected frustrations that one would encounter in interacting with a brain-injured adult.

As a group, the successful patients had significantly less personality, interpersonal, or behavioral difficulty. Table 8.3 illustrates these findings. At the beginning of the NRP (first exam), successful patients were less impaired on all thirteen of the clinical Katz-R Adjustment Scales than were treatment failures. The same pattern held up at the end of the NRP (second exam). Treatment failures generally showed more belligerence, verbal expansiveness, negativism, suspiciousness, signs of general psychopathology, confusion, and lack of social stability.

Three-by-two analyses of variance (i.e., successes vs. intermediates vs. failures × exam 1 vs. exam 2) revealed significance or a trend for significance on the following variables: belligerence ($F = 2.39$, $p = .10$), verbal expansiveness ($F = 5.64$, $p = .0007$), negativism ($F = 3.41$, $p = .04$), general psychopathology ($F = 3.05$, $p = .06$), and instability ($F = 4.59$, $p = .01$). The Duncan Multiple-Range Test generally reflects greater personality and behavioral disturbances in treatment failures versus successes, with intermediates consistently falling between these groups (see Table 8.4). These data reaffirm the clinical impression of the importance of personality variables on the outcome of neuropsychologically oriented rehabilitation.

It has been our clinical impression that patients considered successful not only tended to accept their difficulties but also were generally willing to accept lower levels of employment. This helped them to become more realistic and consequently maintain reasonably good interpersonal relationships. The degree to which the NRP staff fostered these changes was the degree to which it could take credit for substantially aiding the patient and his or her family in the rehabilitation process.

Patients who did not accept their limitations generally had a poor work adjustment. For a patient to become realistic about his or her deficits and to accept life as it is, after exerting considerable effort in the NRP, is no small task, but it is vital to ultimate rehabilitation success. Helping patients forgive themselves and others for what has happened to them may be a crucial element in this regard. Also, the actual amount of brain damage may greatly influence the ability to become aware of and acceptant of cognitive and personality changes after craniocerebral trauma.

Research on the vocational outcome of chronic psychiatric patients has come to essentially the same conclusions (Anthony and Jansen 1984) regarding acceptance and social competency as predictors of employability. The message of this book, as well as the message from previous research on brain-injured patients and psychiatric patients, is clear: if professional rehabilitation staff can help brain-injured patients not alienate others and accept their limitations, major improvements in the rehabilitation outcome of brain-injured patients can occur.

APPENDIX A
Patient Competency Rating (Patient's Form), Neuropsychological Rehabilitation Program, Presbyterian Hospital

Identifying Information

Patient's Name: _____

Patient's Age: _____

Date: _____

Instructions

The following is a questionnaire that asks you to judge your ability to do a variety of very practical skills. Some of the questions may not apply directly to things you often do, but you are asked to complete each question as if it were something you "had to do." On each question, you should judge how easy or difficult a particular activity is for you and mark the appropriate space.

Competency Rating

	Can't do	Very difficult to do	Can do with some difficulty	Fairly easy to do	Can do with ease
1. How much of a problem do I have in preparing my own meals?	___	___	___	___	___
2. How much of a problem do I have in dressing myself?	___	___	___	___	___

	Can't do	Very difficult to do	Can do with some difficulty	Fairly easy to do	Can do with ease
3. How much of a problem do I have in taking care of my personal hygiene?	___	___	___	___	___
4. How much of a problem do I have in washing the dishes?	___	___	___	___	___
5. How much of a problem do I have in doing the laundry?	___	___	___	___	___
6. How much of a problem do I have in taking care of my finances?	___	___	___	___	___
7. How much of a problem do I have in keeping appointments on time?	___	___	___	___	___
8. How much of a problem do I have in starting conversation in a group?	___	___	___	___	___
9. How much of a problem do I have in staying involved in work activities even when bored or tired?	___	___	___	___	___
10. How much of a problem do I have in remembering what I had for dinner last night?	___	___	___	___	___
11. How much of a problem do I have in remembering names of people I see often?	___	___	___	___	___
12. How much of a problem do I have in remembering my daily schedule?	___	___	___	___	___
13. How much of a problem do I have in remembering important things I must do?	___	___	___	___	___

Appendix A   145

	Can't do	Very difficult to do	Can do with some difficulty	Fairly easy to do	Can do with ease
14. How much of a problem would I have driving a car if I had to?	___	___	___	___	___
15. How much of a problem do I have in getting help when I'm confused?	___	___	___	___	___
16. How much of a problem do I have in adjusting to unexpected changes?	___	___	___	___	___
17. How much of a problem do I have in handling arguments with people I know well?	___	___	___	___	___
18. How much of a problem do I have in accepting criticism from other people?	___	___	___	___	___
19. How much of a problem do I have in controlling crying?	___	___	___	___	___
20. How much of a problem do I have in acting appropriately when I'm around friends?	___	___	___	___	___
21. How much of a problem do I have in showing affection to people?	___	___	___	___	___
22. How much of a problem do I have in participating in group activities?	___	___	___	___	___
23. How much of a problem do I have in recognizing when something I say or do has upset someone else?	___	___	___	___	___

	Can't do	Very difficult to do	Can do with some difficulty	Fairly easy to do	Can do with ease
24. How much of a problem do I have in scheduling daily activities?	___	___	___	___	___
25. How much of a problem do I have in understanding new instructions?	___	___	___	___	___
26. How much of a problem do I have in consistently meeting my daily responsibilities?	___	___	___	___	___
27. How much of a problem do I have in controlling my temper when something upsets me?	___	___	___	___	___
28. How much of a problem do I have in keeping from being depressed?	___	___	___	___	___
29. How much of a problem do I have in keeping my emotions from affecting my ability to go about the day's activities?	___	___	___	___	___
30. How much of a problem do I have in controlling my laughter?	___	___	___	___	___

APPENDIX **B**
Patient Competency Rating (Relative's Form), Neuropsychological Rehabilitation Program, Presbyterian Hospital

Patient's Name: _____

Patient's Age: _____

Date: _____

Informant's relationship to patient (circle one):
1. Mother
2. Father
3. Spouse
4. Child
5. Sibling
6. Grandparent
7. Aunt or uncle
8. Niece or nephew
9. Cousin
10. Friend
11. In-law
12. Ward attendant
13. Other _____

Sex of informant:
Male _____
Female _____

How well is informant acquainted with patient's behavior?
1. Hardly at all
2. Not so well
3. Fairly well
4. Pretty well
5. Very well

Instructions

The following is a questionnaire that asks you to judge this person's ability to do a variety of very practical skills. Some of the questions may not apply directly to things they often do, but you are asked to complete each question as if it were something they "had to do." On each question, you should judge how easy or difficult a particular activity is for them and mark the appropriate space.

Competency Rating

	Can't do	Very difficult to do	Can do with some difficulty	Fairly easy to do	Can do with ease
1. How much of a problem do they have in preparing their own meals?	___	___	___	___	___
2. How much of a problem do they have in dressing themselves?	___	___	___	___	___
3. How much of a problem do they have in taking care of their personal hygiene?	___	___	___	___	___
4. How much of a problem do they have in washing the dishes?	___	___	___	___	___
5. How much of a problem do they have in doing the laundry?	___	___	___	___	___
6. How much of a problem do they have in taking care of their finances?	___	___	___	___	___
7. How much of a problem do they have in keeping appointments on time?	___	___	___	___	___
8. How much of a problem do they have in starting conversation in a group?	___	___	___	___	___
9. How much of a problem do they have in staying involved in work activities even when bored or tired?	___	___	___	___	___

	Can't do	Very difficult to do	Can do with some difficulty	Fairly easy to do	Can do with ease
10. How much of a problem do they have in remembering what they had for dinner last night?	——	——	——	——	——
11. How much of a problem do they have in remembering names of people they see often?	——	——	——	——	——
12. How much of a problem do they have in remembering their daily schedule?	——	——	——	——	——
13. How much of a problem do they have in remembering important things they must do?	——	——	——	——	——
14. How much of a problem would they have driving a car if they had to?	——	——	——	——	——
15. How much of a problem do they have in getting help when they are confused?	——	——	——	——	——
16. How much of a problem do they have in adjusting to unexpected changes?	——	——	——	——	——
17. How much of a problem do they have in handling arguments with people they know well?	——	——	——	——	——
18. How much of a problem do they have in accepting criticism from other people?	——	——	——	——	——

150 *Appendix B*

	Can't do	Very difficult to do	Can do with some difficulty	Fairly easy to do	Can do with ease
19. How much of a problem do they have in controlling crying?	___	___	___	___	___
20. How much of a problem do they have in acting appropriately when they are around friends?	___	___	___	___	___
21. How much of a problem do they have in showing affection to people?	___	___	___	___	___
22. How much of a problem do they have in participating in group activities?	___	___	___	___	___
23. How much of a problem do they have in recognizing when something they say or do has upset someone else?	___	___	___	___	___
24. How much of a problem do they have in scheduling daily activities?	___	___	___	___	___
25. How much of a problem do they have in understanding new instructions?	___	___	___	___	___
26. How much of a problem do they have in consistently meeting their daily responsibilities?	___	___	___	___	___
27. How much of a problem do they have in controlling their temper when something upsets them?	___	___	___	___	___
28. How much of a problem do they have in keeping from being depressed?	___	___	___	___	___

	Can't do	Very difficult to do	Can do with some difficulty	Fairly easy to do	Can do with ease
29. How much of a problem do they have in keeping their emotions from affecting their ability to go about the day's activities?	___	___	___	___	___
30. How much of a problem do they have in controlling their laughter?	___	___	___	___	___

APPENDIX C
Revisions to the Neuropsychological Rehabilitation Program at Presbyterian Hospital

From 1980 to 1984 the Neuropsychological Rehabilitation Program at Presbyterian Hospital in Oklahoma City provided a structured daily rehabilitation experience whereby young adult brain-injured patients could come to grips with their cognitive and personality disturbances following brain injury. As a result of that work, we have been impressed with the importance of including an actual work trial as a part of the rehabilitation program. We also discovered that there were some patients who either did not need all the neuropsychological rehabilitation activities originally provided or were unable to profit substantially from them. Consequently, we have revised our program to include a work trial and to allow for greater individual responsiveness to the various patients seeking such services.

Purposes of the Neuropsychological Rehabilitation Program
1. To identify and attempt remediation and/or compensation of cognitive, perceptual, motor, language, personality, and residual physical problems secondary to brain injury
2. To identify and attempt to change behaviors that have a negative impact on work and interpersonal relationships
3. To help patients become aware of and acceptant of those neuropsychological consequences of brain injury that may not change over time and treatment
4. To help patients improve their personal reactions to brain injury
5. To help patients identify, obtain, and/or maintain employment commensurate with their abilities following brain injury

Examples of Problem Areas Addressed in the Neuropsychological Rehabilitation Program
1. Helping patients understand their problems in abstract reasoning and how these lead to overreaction in interpersonal situations

2. Helping patients recognize when they are tangential in their thoughts and communication
3. Helping patients compensate for memory difficulties
4. Helping patients recognize residual strengths and raise self-esteem
5. Helping patients accept the level of employment that will be practical for them (includes dealing with their emotional reactions to loss of former function, status, and income)
6. Helping patients go to work (when it is possible) even when there is a personal or financial pull to stay economically dependent
7. Helping families become realistic about patients' strengths and weaknesses
8. Helping families with their personal reactions or sense of loss over the change in a brain-injured relative
9. Teaching patients how to compare and discuss their views with others without becoming irritated or overreacting emotionally
10. Helping patients identify which motor problems (and language and communication skills) will improve with practice and which will have to be adapted to, especially as relates to work
11. Helping patients recognize that they may process information at a slower rate than they did prior to injury and that they consequently need to learn methods to compensate for this
12. Helping patients learn to become generally more tolerant and less irritable in social situations
13. Helping patients learn strategies for being more efficient, self-starting, and organized in their daily behavior
14. Helping patients realize that they are not alone in their struggle to cope with their brain injury
15. Helping patients realize that facing the tragedy of brain injury in their life can actually provide a basis for more mature interpersonal functioning

Practical Considerations in Doing Neuropsychological Rehabilitation

Young adults who suffer brain injury experience cognitive dysfunction and changes in personality. Sometimes patients are aware of these difficulties, but many times they do not fully appreciate the extent of their problems. Family members and employers try to be supportive and fair, but they are often seen by patients as demanding, nonunderstanding, and manipulative. In response, family members frequently see the patient as selfish, argumentative, unreliable, withdrawn, and unwilling to accept the limitations produced by the brain damage. From this emerge major emotional and motivational disturbances that can further threaten a patient's social support systems. When this happens in a family where the patient and/or family member(s) have preexisting problems in coping with life (i.e., psychiatric disturbances), the rehabilitation process becomes extremely difficult and demanding.

To help patients and their family members understand what is wrong and what realistic steps can be taken in a given patient's care, the patient and family must work in a collaborative effort with the professional rehabilitation team. This includes, by its nature, individual and small-group education and retraining activities.

Individual attention is needed because the brain dysfunctional patient's problems are exceedingly complex and require constant monitoring, evaluation, and intervention. The patient's individual problems, however, influence his or her ability to adapt socially to the environment. Therefore, the patient must also be treated within the context of a social milieu. This can be accomplished only if the rehabilitation involves small-group activities. Likewise, family members need a combination of individual and small-group educational experiences to help them understand the problems of a brain-injured relative and how they may be helping or hurting the rehabilitation process.

The degree of rehabilitation effort put into any given patient is dependent on many factors. First, and most important, is the patient's capacity and willingness to work aggressively at neuropsychological rehabilitation. A second factor is the ability of the rehabilitation staff to understand the patients' difficulties in adapting and to develop a method of rehabilitation that motivates patients to participate. A third factor is the question of the cost-efficiency of rehabilitation. For any given patient the benefit of extensive rehabilitation work versus limited rehabilitation work must be considered in terms of its financial cost. While this is not the most humanitarian consideration, it is an important one. Providing a rehabilitation system that both patients and hospitals can afford is vital if one is to maintain any viable rehabilitation facility.

Services Provided

1. Cognitive retraining: individual and group formats
2. Psychotherapy: individual and group formats
3. Physical therapy
4. Speech and language therapy
5. Occupational therapy
6. Work trial/vocational counseling

A detailed description of these services is provided below (pp. 159–63).

Types of Patients Considered Appropriate for the NRP

Patients should be young adults (sixteen to forty or more years) who have a history of reasonably good personal adjustment prior to their brain injury. They should be relatively free from major psychiatric illness but suffer significant neuropsychological impairments that interfere with their ability to function in a productive and independent fashion. They should have some basic motivation to work at becoming aware of their deficits and be willing to try to compensate for the neuropsychological problems they experience. While such patients may have additional neurological deficits (e.g., motor and perceptual difficulties), they need to have sufficiently good language skills to communicate within group activities. Finally, these patients must have a social support system that encourages them to return to partial or gainful employment. This includes family members who are willing to become actively involved in the rehabilitation process.

The Philosophy of the Program

To achieve the rehabilitation goals set forth for each patient, a sense of mutual cooperation and trust between patients, relatives, and staff is sought. This alliance is crucial for shifting the patient from being a dependent, convalescing person to being a more fully functioning, independent individual. Without a feeling of reciprocal trust and commitment, the fear, anger, depression, and other strong emotions that arise during rehabilitation can be expressed in counterproductive ways. Lack of attendance, uncooperativeness, or violent outbursts are examples of serious problems that can arise. The feelings that underlie these problems are natural reactions to brain injury as well as to the rehabilitation process. The need for patients to assume increasing levels of responsibility for their rehabilitation and personal lives can be particularly frightening. These strong feelings can lead to behaviors that may jeopardize the patient's success as well as that of others in the program. It is hoped that during individual psychotherapy, family counseling, and group psychotherapy sessions patients will learn to manage these feelings.

The program guidelines set forth here were designed to facilitate this sense of cooperation and trust. Successful rehabilitation depends on the commitment of staff, patients, and relatives. Active participation in relatives' groups and family meetings is necessary for a patient's rehabilitation process.

Program Format: Daily Schedule

The Neuropsychological Rehabilitation Program is designed to allow for two major areas of rehabilitation emphasis. Morning hours are devoted to the remediation of and compensation for changes in cognitive, personality, and physical functioning secondary to the brain injury. Afternoon hours are directed toward work trial experiences that help the patient recognize strengths and limitations that must be dealt with if independence in functioning is to be a reality.

8:20–9:00	Cognitive Retraining
9:00–9:40	Individual Therapies
9:40–9:50	Break
9:50–10:30	Cognitive Group
10:30–11:10	Individual Therapies
11:10–11:20	Break
11:20–12:00	Group Psychotherapy
12:00–12:20	Milieu
12:20–1:00	Lunch
1:00–5:00	Work Trial
4:30–5:15 *	Staff Meeting
5:00–6:00	Relatives' Group (Wednesdays)

The Work Trial Program

The work trial program is a new venture for us and has been outlined in "stages."

STAGE I

In Stage I the patient does supervised volunteer work at different work stations within Presbyterian Hospital or other designated area. The patient is evaluated regarding basic work skills and his or her ability to interact effectively with fellow employees. During the first one to two weeks, the NRP staff work side by side with the patient and the job supervisor on the work site to help with initial adjustment and to develop a clear understanding of job duties and responsibilities. This degree of in-person supervision is gradually phased out, so that by the third week telephone calls or in-person visits are made as needed. Information is fed back into the NRP so that the patient can improve basic work competency skills and learn to accept the level of present employment. On successful completion of this stage, the patient will then move to Stage II. We expect that Stage I will last no longer than three months.

STAGE II

In Stage II the patient does volunteer work with minimal supervision and limited pay at different work sites in the greater Oklahoma City community. The patient continues in the NRP in the mornings but works in the

---

* On Wednesdays, the Staff Meeting adjourns at 5:00 P.M. so that staff members can conduct the Relatives' Group.

afternoons with minimal supervision. Either NRP staff or hired vocational counselors will initially go to the work sites and talk with employers and fellow workers to ensure that the patient understands and performs job activities adequately. However, less on-the-job training will be provided by NRP staff at this stage, compared with the very close supervision and assistance developing appropriate work skills of Stage I. Again, information concerning job performance is fed back to the NRP program so that this information can be used to help patients with their work adjustment. Following successful completion of Stage II, Stage III will be attempted. Whenever possible, Stage II placements will be made with companies willing to hire brain-injured individuals as regular employees *if* the Stage II trial is successful and all parties involved are interested in a transition to full-time paid employment. Stage II is expected to last from the fourth month through the sixth month.

STAGE III

In Stage III the patient will attempt to find gainful employment in either the Oklahoma City community or in his or her home community, or move from Stage II to Stage III status within the same company. The patient will remain in contact with the NRP staff for a minimum of one to three months to ensure that a successful transition into a gainful employment setting has been accomplished. The patient may or may not be involved in the intensive NRP during this time, but nevertheless will be seen periodically by the NRP staff to ensure that the transition back to work is meaningful and one that the patient can accept and manage.

Some patients may not successfully complete Stage I or Stage II within a six-month period of time, while other patients may work their way more quickly through these stages. Failure to complete Stage I or Stage II successfully within a six-month framework would be used as fairly objective evidence either of rehabilitation failure or that gainful employment is not a realistic goal. The patient, family, and third-party payor will receive monthly statements regarding patient progress.

Monthly Evaluations and Tailoring the Program to Individual Needs

Each month the neuropsychological rehabilitation staff will meet formally and review the patient's progress. At this time they will state in writing the progress and prognosis for gainful employment. Recommendations concerning length of stay in the program will be reevaluated with documentation. Typically, the patient and family will be asked to make a six-month commitment to the program, but depending on the patient's individual needs and progress, this time period may be shortened or lengthened.

Patients will be involved in both individual and group work, but the amount and type of work will depend on individual needs. Furthermore, the individual therapies the patients will receive will be dictated by their progress in the rehabilitation program and the degree to which they show benefit from various activities. All patients will be involved in designated group activities to help deal with the problems of social competency and eventual awareness and acceptance of residual disabilities.

The exact format for each patient's program will be provided in writing to the patient, the insurance carrier, and the family once a patient is accepted into the program. It is felt that this tailoring of the program to each individual patient will allow for greater flexibility in terms of our work commitment to patients and their understanding of what is required of them during their participation in the program.

Initial Referral and Evaluation

Patients who seek entry into the program are first seen for a comprehensive neuropsychological examination or evaluation. That initial referral is frequently made by a physician, psychologist, family member, insurance carrier, attorney, or social agency. After that initial examination-evaluation is done, we attempt to make some initial determination as to whether the patient would be an appropriate candidate for the program. If there is doubt or if more information is needed, one of the other therapists (a speech and language pathologist, occupational therapist, or physical therapist) may be asked to become involved in the evaluation process.

The patient and family are then informed of the findings and recommendations verbally and in writing. In some instances, patients will be asked to be involved on a clinical trial basis in order to determine whether it is appropriate for them to become part of the program.

Financial Considerations

Important financial considerations are the cost of the program to the patient and the steps that can be taken to help patients pay for the rehabilitative services.

THE COST TO THE PATIENT

Intensive daily neuropsychologically oriented rehabilitation is costly from a financial and an emotional point of view, but proper planning can help make these costs manageable. The professional fees vary over time. To keep costs at a minimum, we conduct a *day treatment* program instead of an inpatient program.

FINANCIAL PLANNING

Besides the professional steps necessary to determine if a patient is appropriate for this rehabilitation program, a series of financial steps should be taken to increase the probability of payment for services if the patient is accepted.

Step 1

Once the initial neuropsychological examination is completed and entry into the program is a possibility, *immediately* check with insurance carriers regarding possible coverage for these services. It usually takes several weeks, if not months, to get a definite answer. We suggest that insurance confirmation be obtained in writing.

Step 2

If the insurance carriers indicate they will pay a portion of the costs, *determine* the anticipated benefits, how the bill must be filed, and to whom the bill must be sent. If the insurance carriers will not pay for a portion of the costs, determine other sources of possible financial aid. State vocational rehabilitation services may cover some patients if financial need is determined and if it is clear that the patient has a high likelihood of benefiting. You must contact your local vocational rehabilitation counselor immediately regarding this and work closely to get a definite determination.

Step 3

If there are no external sources of financial support available and the family resources do not allow for direct payment of services as they are incurred, in *selected* cases the Business Office of Presbyterian Hospital will determine whether the patient is eligible for an alternative agreement. Those who may be eligible for an alternative agreement are usually young adults who have suffered brain injury in the midst of professional training or right after gainful employment. If they return to work, they will be able to pay for the services received in the program.

Description of Services

The services provided by the program include individual therapy, group cognitive retraining, cognitive group therapy, group psychotherapy, work trial and vocational counseling, "milieu" (a community group meeting), and a relatives' group.

INDIVIDUAL THERAPY

Individual therapy (cognitive retraining, speech and language therapy, psychotherapy, occupational therapy, and physical therapy) is designed to provide individual treatment specific to the particular needs of each patient. Participation in any given activity is determined by staff observations and discussions between patients and staff regarding areas of most critical intervention.

Cognitive Retraining

Cognitive retraining is a broad term used to refer to a variety of activities aimed at helping a patient improve specific higher cerebral functioning. It includes three basic subtypes:

1. Cognitive-judgment compensation training: a series of training exercises designed to improve the patient's higher-order thinking functions. This includes (a) judgment (common sense), sizing up a situation, comprehension of the "core" or essence of a situation; (b) expressive skills, the ability to clearly convey meanings; (c) recognition of problems, focusing in on a problem; and (d) problem-solving abilities, e.g., use of organizing, planning, and sequencing techniques, the ability to draw correct inferences, and the ability to order behaviors into priorities and to carry through solutions.
2. Perceptual-motor training: remediation techniques consisting of both retraining and compensatory training of hand-eye coordination, finger dexterity, visual-spatial information-processing, visual-constructional, sequential, and integrational skills, facilitating spatial and temporal orientation, sustaining perceptual attention, vigilance, and arousal.
3. Memory compensation training: a series of remediation techniques designed to counter problems of initial registration and learning, as well as retention problems of both short-term and long-term memory deficits. This training attempts to develop efficient information encoding with supplemental techniques to enhance both verbal and nonverbal memory and information-processing.

Physical Therapy

Physical therapy is a form of professional patient care aimed at restoring motor function, relieving pain, and preventing disability following disease, injury, or loss of body part. These services are rendered by a registered physical therapist. For many brain-injured patients, a significant reduction in general physical endurance, fitness, and tone seems to develop with time after the acute recovery phase. Physical therapy intervention helps these patients develop and maintain the basic energy levels needed for productive work and interpersonal functioning.

Speech and Language Therapy

Speech and language therapy is a discipline that deals with diagnosis and treatment of functional and organic disorders of speech and/or language. It stresses both remediation and compensation for specific deficits in communication skills. This service is provided by a certified speech and language pathologist.

Occupational Therapy

Occupational therapy traditionally emphasizes achieving maximal independence in work, leisure, and self-care, but it also further focuses on gross, fine, and perceptual motor activities as well as effective group interaction. Activities are directed toward facilitating memory compensation and appropriate social skills to allow patients to function in their varied environmental settings. Treatment is provided by a registered occupational therapist.

Psychotherapy

Often patients' personal adjustment problems require more than group intervention, and these individuals are seen for individual psychotherapy. At times, some patients experience considerable difficulty with the rehabilitation program and may need individual help to follow through in sustaining their rehabilitation efforts. At other times, the patient simply needs individual psychotherapy to pursue more personalized discussion of issues related to the brain injury.

GROUP COGNITIVE RETRAINING

Activities undertaken during cognitive group retraining focus on three major areas of cognitive functioning that typically are disordered following brain injury: orientation, the speed and efficiency of information-processing, and basic academic skills (i.e., reading, writing, arithmetic). Problems in these areas are so common following brain injury and produce such basic roadblocks to successful rehabilitation that they are stressed intensively in this early morning hour.

Two or three patients will work at an individual table with a single staff member. The staff member will supervise and monitor each patient's individual work in the various cognitive retraining activities. Progress will be charted and regularly reviewed, and new tasks will be introduced when the individual patient reaches maximum performance on the current activity.

The initial focus is on improving orientation and increasing attention span. Later tasks grow more complex and require increased speed and efficiency in performance and the development of problem-solving strategies.

Staffing is provided by a speech and language pathologist, occupational therapist, and/or clinical psychologist.

COGNITIVE GROUP THERAPY

Cognitive group therapy is a form of group therapy that focuses on improving social perceptions and enhancing clear and effective communications. These areas represent major hurdles during the process of social and vocational readjustment and for this reason receive a great deal of attention during cognitive group therapy.

Initially the purpose of the group is to increase the level of self-awareness of residual cognitive strengths and weaknesses. The process frequently generates strong emotional reactions, but it is necessary to help individuals recognize and formulate realistic perceptions of self and environment. This ability is critical and a vital step toward successful rehabilitation.

Later, cognitive group therapy focuses on improving thinking and communication in group settings. Activities are intended to increase organizational skills, logic, and the processes of divergent and convergent thinking. The goal is to reduce tangential thinking and other ineffective communication patterns.

During cognitive group activities it is the responsibility of group members to provide appropriate feedback to one another in a clear and concise fashion. Group interaction is extremely important because it is often easier for patients to see characteristics in others before recognizing the same characteristic in themselves. This requires sustained attention on the part of each participant and a maximum level of participation. This group is led by a speech and language pathologist and a psychologist.

GROUP PSYCHOTHERAPY

Group psychotherapy is a traditional group therapy directed at the emotional and motivational disturbances associated with brain injury. The focus is on helping the patient recognize and face those personality disturbances which are reactionary in nature, those that are neuropsychologically mediated, and others that are characterological or long-term in nature. Patients are helped to understand their different types of affective disturbances associated with their injury. Successful modification of these affective problems is necessary to facilitate the rehabilitation process. This group is conducted by two clinical neuropsychologists.

WORK TRIAL/VOCATIONAL COUNSELING

In work trial and vocational counseling, a full afternoon's activity, volunteer work placements are undertaken by each patient with close assistance and supervision provided by NRP staff. As work readiness skills improve, the patient is expected to function independently in this kind of setting, with minimal NRP staff supervision. During this same period of time, contact will be made with selected professional vocational counselors, who will serve as consultants to the NRP. These vocational counselors will assist NRP staff in obtaining regular work placements for patients. If a patient enters with excellent work skills, his or her initial placement might be in a limited-pay or regular full-time work position. For other patients, time spent in volunteer status and time spent improving work skills will be a major focus. The work trial and vocational counseling part of the program has been designed to allow for individual needs and abilities.

MILIEU

Milieu is a community group meeting involving all the patients and staff in the rehabilitation program. It is held at the end of each rehabilitation day and has as its purpose the discussion of any issues that are related to the smooth operation of the program. These may include attendance problems, friction among group members, patient participation, patient progress, program business, and other issues that arise during the program. This is an important time for patients to discuss these issues openly and to provide or receive appropriate feedback from members of the program.

RELATIVES' GROUP

Relatives' Group is an educational as well as group therapy experience for relatives of the brain-injured. It is aimed at providing objective information to relatives about brain injury and the psychological sequelae. It is also a time to discuss personal reactions in dealing with a brain-injured relative and maximizing their home management. This group is led by two staff members, one of whom is either the director or the co-director of the Neuropsychological Rehabilitation Program.

References

Achenbach, T. M., and Edelbrock, C. S. 1981. Behavioral problems and competencies reported by parents of normal and disturbed children aged four through sixteen. *Monographs of the Society for Research in Child Development 46 (1),* 1–82.

Adams, J. H. 1975. The neuropathology of head injuries. In P. J. Vinken and G. W. Bruyn, eds., *Handbook of Clinical Neurology,* Volume 23. New York: Elsevier–North Holland Publishing Co.

Anthony, W. A., and Jansen, M. A. 1984. Predicting the vocational capacity of the chronically mentally ill. *American Psychologist 39(5),* 537–544.

Bach, S. R. 1969. Spontaneous paintings of severely ill patients: A contribution to psychosomatic medicine. *Acta Psychosomatica,* no. 8. Basle, Switz.: G. R. Geigy.

Baker, G. 1955. Diagnosis of organic brain damage in the adult. In B. Klopfer, ed., *Developments in the Rorschach Technique,* Volume 2. Yonkers-on-Hudson, N.Y.: World Book Co.

Barr, A. J.; Goodnight, J. H.; Sall, P.; and Helwig, J. T., eds. 1976. *A User's Guide to SAS 76.* Raleigh, N.C.: Statistical Analysis System Institute.

Bear, D. M. 1983. Hemispheric specialization and the neurology of emotion *Archives of Neurology 40,* 195–202.

Benson, D. F. 1979. Aphasia. In K. M. Heilman and E. Valenstein, eds., *Clinical Neuropsychology.* New York: Oxford University Press.

Benson, D. F.; Stuss, D. T.; Maeser, M. A.; Weir, W. S.; Kaplan, E. F.; and Levin, H. L. 1981. The long-term effects of prefrontal leukotomy. *Archives of Neurology 38,* 165–169.

Ben-Yishay, Y., and Diller, L. 1981. *Working Approaches to Remediation of Cognitive Deficits in Brain Damage.* Supplement to Ninth Annual Workshop for Rehabilitation Professionals, New York University, Institute of Rehabilitation Medicine.

―――. 1983. Cognitive deficits. In M. Rosenthal, E. Griffith, M. Bond, and J. D. Miller, eds. *Rehabilitation of the Head-injured Adult.* Philadelphia: F. A. Davis Co.

Ben-Yishay, Y.; Diller, L.; Gerstman, L; and Gordon, W. 1970. Relationship between initial competence and ability to profit from cues in brain-damaged individuals. *Journal of Abnormal Psychology 75,* 248-259.

Ben-Yishay, Y.; Diller, L.; Mandleberg, I.; Gordon, W.; and Gerstman, L. 1971. Similarities and differences in block design performance between older normal and brain-injured persons: A task analysis. *Journal of Abnormal Psychology 78,* 17-25.

Ben-Yishay, Y.; Rattok, J.; and Diller, L. 1979. *Working Approaches to Remediation of Cognitive Deficits in Brain Damage.* Supplement to Seventh Annual Workshop for Rehabilitation Professionals, New York University, Institute of Rehabilitation Medicine.

Ben-Yishay, Y.; Rattok, J.; Ross, B.; Lakin, P.; Silver, S.; Thomas, L.; and Diller, L. 1982. *Working Approaches to Remediation of Cognitive Deficits in Brain Damage.* Supplement to Tenth Annual Workshop for Rehabilitation Professionals, New York University, Institute of Rehabilitation Medicine.

Blumer, D., and Benson, D. F. 1975. Personality changes with frontal and temporal lobe lesions. In D. F. Benson and D. Blumer, eds., *Psychiatric Aspects of Neurologic Disease.* New York: Grune and Stratton.

Bond, M. R. 1975. Assessment of the psychosocial outcome after severe head injury. In CIBA Foundation, *Outcome of Severe Damage to the Central Nervous System,* New York: Elsevier-North Holland Publishing Co.

―――. 1983. Effects on the family system. In W. Rosenthal, R. Griffith, M. Bond, and J. D. Miller, eds., *Rehabilitation of the Head-injured Adult.* Philadelphia: F. A. Davis Co.

Bond, M. R., and Brooks, D. N. 1976. Understanding the process of recovery as a basis for the investigation of rehabilitation for the brain injured. *Scandinavian Journal of Rehabilitation Medicine 8,* 127-133.

Braakman, R.; Gelpke, G. J.; Habbema, J.D.F.; Maas, A.I.P.; and Minderhoud, J. M. 1980. Systematic selection of features in patients with severe head injury. *Neurosurgery 6,* 362-370.

Brooks, D. N. 1983. Disorders of memory. In W. Rosenthal, R. Griffith, M. Bond, and J. D. Miller, eds., *Rehabilitation of the Head-injured Adult.* Philadelphia: F. A. Davis Co.

Brown, G.; Chadwick, O.; Shaffer, D.; Rutter, M.; and Traub, M. 1981. A prospective study of children with head injuries, III: Psychiatric sequelae. *Psychological Medicine 11,* 63-78.

Bruckner, F. E., and Randle, A.P.H. 1972. Return to work after severe head injuries. *Rheumatology and Physical Medicine 11,* 344-348.

Buss, A. H. 1966. *Psychopathology.* New York: John Wiley and Sons.

Butters, N. 1979. Amnestic disorders. In K. M. Heilman and E. Valenstein, eds., *Clinical Neuropsychology.* New York: Oxford University Press.

Chadwick, O.; Rutter, M.; Brown, G.; Shaffer, D.; and Traub, M. 1981. A prospective study of children with head injuries, II: Cognitive sequelae. *Psychological Medicine 11,* 49-61.

Cummings, N. A. 1977. The anatomy of psychotherapy under national health insurance. *American Psychologist 32,* 711-718.

Curtis, B. A.; Jacobson, S.; and Marcus, E. M. 1972. *An Introduction to the Neurosciences.* Philadelphia: W. B. Saunders Co.

Darley, F. L. 1972. The efficacy of language rehabilitation in aphasia. *Journal of Speech Hearing Disorders 30,* 3-22.

Dean, Paul. 1984. An oasis of hope for the handicapped is blooming in the Arizona desert. *Los Angeles Times,* January 3.

Dennerll, R. D.; Rodin, E. A.; Gonzalez, S.; Schwartz, M. L.,; and Lin, Y. 1966. Neurological and psychological factors related to employability of persons with epilepsy. *Epilepsia 7,* 318-329.

Dikmen, S., and Morgan, S. F. 1980. Neuropsychological factors related to employability and occupational status in persons with epilepsy. *Journal of Nervous and Mental Diseases 168(4),* 236-240.

Dikmen, S., and Reitan, R. M. 1977. MMPI correlates of adaptive ability deficits in patients with brain lesions. *Journal of Nervous and Mental Diseases 165,* 247-253.

Diller, L. 1976. A model for cognitive retraining in rehabilitation. *The Clinical Psychologist 29,* 13-15.

Diller, L.; Ben-Yishay, Y.; Weinberg, J.; Goodkin, R.; and Gordon, W. 1974. Studies in cognition and rehabilitation in hemiplegia. *New York University Medical Center Rehabilitation Monograph 50.* New York: NYU Medical Center.

Diller, L., and Gordon, W. A. 1981. Interventions for cognitive deficits in brain-injured adults. *Journal of Consulting and Clinical Psychology 49,* 822-834.

Dresser, A. C.; Meirowsky, A. M.; Weiss, G. H.; McNeel, M. L.; Simon, G. A.; and Caveness, W. F. 1973. Gainful employment following head injury. *Archives of Neurology 29,* 111-116.

Eccles, J. C. 1977. *The Understanding of the Brain.* New York: McGraw-Hill.

Fahy, T. J.; Irving, M. H.; and Millac, P. 1967. Severe head injuries. *Lancet 2,* 475-479.

Ferguson, S. M.; Schwartz, M. L.; and Rayport, M. 1969. Perception of humor in patients with temporal lobe epilepsy. *Archives of General Psychiatry 21,* 363-367.

Fingers, S., ed. 1978. *Recovery from Brain Injury.* New York: Plenum Press.

Finklestein, S.; Benowitz, L.; Baldessarini, R.; Arana, G.; Levine, D.; Woo, E.; Bear, D.; Moya, K.; and Stoll, A. 1982. Mood, vegetative disturbance, and dexamethasone suppression test after stroke. *Annals of Neurology 12,* 463-468.

Flavell, J. H. 1977. *Cognitive Development.* Englewood Cliffs, N.J.: Prentice-Hall.

Fordyce, D. J. 1983. Underestimates of behavioral dysfunction in brain-injured individuals: Assessment methodology and implications for rehabilitation and psychosocial adjustment. Paper presented at the Third International Symposium on Models and Techniques of Cognitive Rehabilitation, Indianapolis, Ind., March 25-30.

Fordyce, D. J.; Roueche, J. R.; and Prigatano, G. P. 1983. Enhanced emotional reactions in chronic head trauma patients. *Journal of Neurology, Neurosurgery, and Psychiatry 46,* 620-624.

Freedman, A. M.; Kaplan, H. I.; and Sadock, B. J. 1976. *Modern Synopsis of Comprehensive Textbook of Psychiatry,* Second Edition. Baltimore: Williams and Wilkins.

Freud, S. 1924. *A General Introduction to Psychoanalysis,* Twenty-fourth Edition. New York: Simon and Schuster.

Fuster, J. M. 1980. *The Prefrontal Cortex.* New York: Raven Press.
Gainotti, G. 1972. Emotional behavior and hemispheric side of lesion. *Cortex 8,* 41–55.
Gans, J. S. 1983. Hate in the rehabilitation setting. *Archives of Physical Medicine and Rehabilitation 64,* 176–179.
Gasparrini, B., and Satz, P. 1979. A treatment for memory problems in left hemisphere CVA patients. *Journal of Clinical Neuropsychology 1,* 137–150.
Gazzaniga, M. S. 1978. Is seeing believing: Notes on clinical recovery. In S. Finger, ed., *Recovery from Brain Damage.* New York: Plenum Press.
Geschwind, N. 1964. Nonaphasic disorders of speech. *International Journal of Neurology 4,* 207–214.
Gianutsos, R., and Gianutsos, J. 1979. Rehabilitating the verbal recall of brain injured patients by mnemonic training: An experimental demonstration using single case methodology. *Journal of Clinical Neuropsychology 1,* 117–136.
Gilchrist, E., and Wilkinson, M. 1979. Some factors determining prognosis in young people with severe head injuries. *Archives of Neurology 36,* 355–358.
Goldstein, K. 1942. *Aftereffects of Brain Injury in War.* New York: Grune and Stratton.
———. 1952. The effect of brain damage on the personality. *Psychiatry 15,* 245–260.
Graham, D. I.; Adams, J. H.; and Doyle, D. 1978. Ischemic brain damage in fatal nonmissile head injuries. *Journal of Neurological Sciences 39,* 213–234.
Green, P. E. 1978. *Analyzing Multivariate Data.* Hinsdale, Ill.: Dryden Press.
Gronwall, D., and Sampson, H. 1974. *The Psychological Effects of Concussion.* New Zealand: Auckland University Press.
Gronwall, D., and Wrightson, P. 1981. Memory and information processing capacity after closed head injury. *Journal of Neurology, Neurosurgery, and Psychiatry 44,* 889–895.
Halstead, W. C. 1947. *Brain and Intelligence.* Chicago: University of Chicago Press.
Heaton, R. K.; Chelune, G. J.; and Lehman, R.A.W. 1978. Using neuropsychological and personality tests to assess the likelihood of patient employment. *Journal of Nervous and Mental Disease 166(6),* 408–416.
Heaton, R. K., and Pendleton, M. T. 1981. Use of neuropsychological tests to predict adult patients' everyday functioning. *Journal of Consulting and Clinical Psychology 49,* 807–821.
Heilman, K. M. 1979. Neglect and related disorders. In K. M. Heilman and E. Valenstein, eds., *Clinical Neuropsychology.* New York: Oxford University Press.
Hogarty, G. E., and Katz, M. M. 1971. Norms of adjustment and social behavior. *Archives of General Psychiatry 25,* 470–480.
Jennett, B. 1978. If my son had a head injury. *British Medical Journal 1,* 1601–1603.
Jennett, B.; Teasdale, G.; Galbraith, S.; Pickard, J.; Grant, H.; Braakman, R; Avezaat, C.; Maas, A.; Minderhoud, J.; Vecht, F.; Heiden, J.; Small, R.; Caton, W.; and Kurze, T. 1977. Severe head injuries in three countries. *Journal of Neurology, Neurosurgery, and Psychiatry 40,* 291–298.

Jung, C. G. 1964. *Man and His Symbols.* Garden City, N.Y.: Doubleday/Windfall.
Kertesz, A., and McCabe, P. 1977. Recovery patterns and prognosis in aphasia. *Brain 100,* 1–18.
Kinsbourne, M. 1971. The minor cerebral hemisphere as a source of aphasic speech. *Archives of Neurology 25,* 302–306.
Kozol, H. L. 1945. Pretraumatic personality and psychiatric sequelae of head injury. *Archives of Neurology and Psychiatry 53,* 358–364.
———. 1946. Pretraumatic personality and psychiatric sequelae of head injury. *Archives of Neurology and Psychiatry 56,* 245–275.
Kuffler, S. W., and Nicholls, J. G. 1977. *From Neuron to Brain.* Sunderland, Mass.: Sinauer Associates.
Kun, L. E.; Mulhern, R. K.; and Crisco, J. J. 1983. Quality of life in children treated for brain tumors. *Journal of Neurosurgery 58,* 1–6.
Labaw, W. 1969. Denial inside out: Subjective experiences with anosognosia in closed head injury. *Psychiatry 32,* 174–191.
Lackner, J. R. 1974. Observations on the speech processing capabilities of an amnestic patient: Several aspects of H.M.'s language function. *Neuropsychologia 12,* 199–207.
———. 1982. Alterations and resolution of linguistic ambiguity after cerebral injury in man. *Perceptual and Motor Skills 54,* 283–289.
Lazarus, R. S. 1977. Psychological stress and coping in adaptation and illness. In Z. J. Lipowski, D. R. Lipsitt, and P. C. Whyleron, eds., *Psychosomatic Medicine: Current Trends and Applications.* New York: Oxford University Press.
Leftoff, S. 1983. Psychopathology in the light of brain injury: A case study. *Journal of Clinical Neuropsychology 5(1),* 51–63.
Levin, H. S.; Benton, A. L.; and Grossman, R. G. 1983. *Neurobehavioral Consequences of Closed Head Injury.* New York: Oxford University Press.
Levin, H. S., and Grossman, R. G. 1978. Behavioral sequelae of closed head injury: A quantitative study. *Archives of Neurology 35,* 720–727.
Levin, H. S.; Grossman, R. G.; and Kelly, P. J. 1976. Aphasic disorder in patients with closed head injury. *Journal of Neurology, Neurosurgery, and Psychiatry 39,* 1062–1070.
Levin, H. S.; Grossman, R. G., Rose, J. E.; and Teasdale, G. 1979. Long-term neuropsychological outcome of closed head injury. *Journal of Neurosurgery 50,* 412–422.
Levin, H. S.; Grossman, R. G.; Sarwar, M.; and Meyers, C. A. 1981. Linguistic recovery after closed head injury. *Brain and Language 12,* 360–374.
Lewin, W. N.; Marshall, T. F.; and Roberts, A. H. 1979. Long-term outcome after severe head injury. *British Medical Journal 2,* 1533–1538.
Lezak, M. D. 1978. Living with the characterologically altered brain-injured patient. *Journal of Clinical Psychiatry 39(7),* 592–598.
Lindsley, D. B. 1970. The role of nonspecific reticulo-thalamocortical systems in emotion. In P. Black, ed., *Physiological Correlates of Emotion.* New York: Academic Press.
Lipper, S., and Tuchman, M. M. 1976. Treatment of chronic posttraumatic or-

ganic brain syndrome with dextroamphetamine: First reported case. *Journal of Nervous and Mental Diseases 162(5),* 366-371.

Lipton, M. A.; Dimascio, A.; and Killam, K. F., eds. 1978. *Psychopharmacology: A Generation of Progress.* New York: Raven Press.

Lishman, W. A. 1968. Brain damage in relation to psychiatric disability after head injury. *British Journal of Psychiatry 114,* 373-410.

———. 1973. The psychiatric sequelae of head injury: A review. *Psychological Medicine 3,* 304-318.

Lorenz, K. 1966. *On Aggression.* New York: Harcourt, Brace and World.

Luria, A. R. 1948. *Restoration of Functions After Brain Trauma* (in Russian). Moscow: Academy of Medical Science Press. London: Pergamon Press, 1963.

———. 1966. *Higher Cortical Functions in Man.* New York: Basic Books.

———. 1977. *Neuropsychological Studies in Aphasia.* Amsterdam: Swets and Zeitlinger.

Luria, A. R.; Naydin, V. L.; Tsvetkova, L. W.; and Vinarskava, E. N. 1969. Restoration of higher cortical function following local brain damage. In P. J. Vinken and G. W. Bruyn, eds., *Handbook of Clinical Neurology,* Volume 3. New York: Elsevier-North Holland Publishing Co.

Mandleberg, I. A., and Brooks, D. N. 1975. Cognitive recovery after severe head injury, I: Serial testing on the Wechsler Adult Intelligence Scale. *Journal of Neurology, Neurosurgery, and Psychiatry 38,* 1121-1126.

Marin, O. S.; Schwartz, M. F.; and Saffran, E. M. 1979. Origins and distribution of language. In M. S. Gazzaniga, ed., *Handbook of Behavioral Neurobiology,* Volume 2. New York: Plenum Press.

Mash, E. J., and Johnston, C. 1983. Parental perceptions of child behavior problems, parenting self-esteem, and mothers' reported stress in younger and older hyperactive and normal children. *Journal of Consulting and Clinical Psychology 51(1),* 86-99.

McLean, A.; Temkin, N. R.; Dikmen, S.; and Wyler, A. R. 1983. The behavior sequelae of minor head injury. *Journal of Clinical Neuropsychology.*

McSweeny, A. R.; Grant, I.; Heaton, R. K.; Adams, K. M.; and Timms, R. M. 1982. Life quality of patients with chronic obstructive pulmonary disease. *Archives of Internal Medicine 142(4),* 473-478.

Miller, E. 1980. The training characteristics of severely head-injured patients: A preliminary study. *Journal of Neurology, Neurosurgery, and Psychiatry 43,* 525-528.

Miller, G. A.; Galanter, E.; and Pribram, K. H. 1960. *Plans and the Structure of Behavior.* New York: Holt, Rinehart, and Winston.

Morrow, L.; Vrtunski, K.; Kim, Y.; and Boller, F. 1981. Arousal responses to emotional stimuli and laterality of lesion. *Neuropsychologia 19,* 65-71.

Najenson, T.; Mendelson, L.; Schechter, I.; David, C.; Mintz, N.; and Groswasser, Z. 1976. Rehabilitation after severe head injury. *Scandinavian Journal of Rehabilitation Medicine 6,* 5-14.

Newcombe, F. 1969. *Missile Wounds of the Brain.* New York: Oxford University Press.

Newcombe, F., and Ratcliff, G. 1979. Long-term psychological consequences of cerebral lesions. In M. S. Gazzaniga, ed., *Handbook of Behavioral Neurobiology*, Volume 2. New York: Plenum Press.

Newnan, O. S.; Heaton, R. K.; and Lehman, A. W. 1978. Neuropsychological and MMPI correlates of patients' future employment characteristics. *Perceptual and Motor Skills 46*, 635–642.

Oddy, M.; Humphrey, M.; and Uttley, D. 1978a. Subjective impairment and social recovery after closed head injury. *Journal of Neurology, Neurosurgery, and Psychiatry 41*, 611–616.

———. 1978b. Stresses upon the relatives of head injured patients. *British Journal of Psychiatry 133*, 507–513.

Ommaya, A. K., and Gennarelli, T. A. 1974. Cerebral concussion and unconsciousness: Correlation of experimental and clinical observations on blunt head injuries. *Brain 97*, 633–654.

Parsons, O. A., and Prigatano, G. P. 1978. Methodological considerations in clinical neuropsychological research. *Journal of Consulting and Clinical Psychology 46*, 608–619.

Poeck, K. 1969. Pathophysiology of emotional disorders associated with brain damage. In P. J. Vinken and A. W. Bruyn, eds., *Handbook of Clinical Neurology*, Volume 3. New York: Elsevier–North Holland Publishing Co.

Pribram, K. H. 1971. *Languages of the Brain: Experimental Paradoxes and Principles in Neuropsychology*, Second Edition. Englewood Cliffs, N.J.: Prentice-Hall.

———. 1977. New dimensions in the function of basal ganglia. In C. Shagass, S. Gershen, and A. J. Friedhoff, eds., *Psychopathology and Brain Dysfunction*. New York: Raven Press.

Pribram, K. H., and Gill, M. M. 1976. *Freud's "Project" Reassessed*. New York: Basic Books.

Pribram, K. H., and Luria, A. R., eds. 1973. *Psychophysiology of the Frontal Lobes*. New York: Academic Press.

Pribram, K. H., and McGuinness, D. 1975. Arousal, activation, and effect in the control of attention. *Psychological Review 82*, 116–149.

Prigatano, G. P. 1978. The Wechsler Memory Scale: A selective review of the literature. *Journal of Clinical Psychology 34(4)*, 816–832; and *Archives of the Behavioral Sciences, Monograph 54*, October.

———. 1981. Dealing with the emotional-motivational disturbances of the traumatic head injury patient. Invited symposium on Rehabilitation of Post-traumatic Brain Damaged Patients, American Psychological Association Convention, Los Angeles.

———. 1983a. Visual imagery and the corpus callosum: A theoretical note. *Perceptual and Motor Skills 56*, 296–298.

———. 1983b. The role of cognition as it affects psychosocial adjustment. Paper presented at the Third International Symposium on Models and Techniques of Cognitive Rehabilitation, Indianapolis, Ind., March 25–30.

———. In press. Personality and psychosocial consequences after brain injury. In M. Meier, L. Diller, and A. Benton, eds., *Neuropsychological Rehabilitation*. London: Churchill Livingstone.

Prigatano, G. P., and Fordyce, D. J. In press. Neuropsychological rehabilitation program. In B. Caplan and G. Bray, eds., *Handbook of Contemporary Rehabilitation Psychology*. Springfield, Ill.: Charles C Thomas Publishing Co.

Prigatano, G. P.; Fordyce, D. J.; Zeiner, H. K.; Roueche, J. R.; Pepping, M.; and Wood, B. 1983. Neuropsychological rehabilitation of closed head injury patients. Paper presented at the International Conference on Management of Traumatic Brain Injury, London, July 14–16.

———. 1984. Neuropsychological rehabilitation after closed head injury in young adults. *Journal of Neurology, Neurosurgery, and Psychiatry 47,* 505–513.

Prigatano, G. P.; Parsons, O. A.; Wright, E.; Levin, D. P.; and Hawryluk, G. 1983. Neuropsychological test performance in mildly hypoxemic patients with chronic obstructive pulmonary disease. *Journal of Consulting and Clinical Psychology 51,* 108–116.

Prigatano, G. P., and Pribram, K. H. 1981. Humor and episodic memory following frontal versus posterior brain lesion. *Perceptual and Motor Skills 53,* 999–1006.

———. 1982. Perception and memory of facial affect following brain injury. *Perceptual and Motor Skills 54,* 859–869.

Prigatano, G. P.; Roueche, J. R.; and Fordyce, D. J. In press. Nonaphasic language disturbances in chronic head trauma patients. In F.C.C. Peng, ed., *Language Sciences* monograph.

Prigatano, G. P.; Stahl, M. L.; Orr, W. C.; and Zeiner, H. K. 1982. Sleep and dreaming disturbances in closed head injury patients. *Journal of Neurology, Neurosurgery, and Psychiatry 45,* 78–80.

Prigatano, G. P., and Zeiner, H. K. In press. Information processing and reading competencies in hydrocephalic and letter reversal children. In F.C.C. Peng, ed., *Neurology of Languages: A First Approximation.* London: Lawrence Erlbaum Associates.

Reitan, R. M. 1952. Affective disturbances in brain-damaged patients. *Archives of Neurology and Psychiatry 73,* 530–532.

Reitan, R. M., and Davison, L. 1974. *Clinical Neuropsychology: Current Status and Applications.* New York: John Wiley and Sons.

Rimel, R. W.; Giordani, B.; Barth, J. T.; Boll, T. J.; and Jane, J. A. 1981. Disability caused by minor head injury. *Neurosurgery 9(3),* 221–228.

Rimel, R. W.; Giordani, B.; Barth, J. T.; and Jane, J. A. 1982. Moderate head injury: Completing the clinical spectrum of brain trauma. *Neurosurgery 11(3),* 344–350.

Roberts, A. H. 1979. *Severe Accidental Head Injury.* London: Macmillan.

Rochester, S. R.; Martin, J. R.; and Thurston, S. 1977. Thought process disorder in schizophrenia: The listener's task. *Brain and Language 4,* 95–114.

Romano, M. D. 1974. Family response to traumatic head injury. *Scandinavian Journal of Rehabilitation Medicine 6,* 1–4.

Rosenbaum, M.; Lipsitz, N.; Abraham, J.; and Najenson, T. 1978. A description of an intensive treatment project for the rehabilitation of severely brain-injured patients. *Scandinavian Journal of Rehabilitative Medicine 10,* 1–6.

Rosenthal, M.; Griffith, E.; Bond, M.; and Miller, J. D., eds. 1983. *Rehabilitation of the Head Injured Adult.* Philadelphia: F. A. Davis.

Roueche, J. R., and Fordyce, D. J. 1983. Perceptions of deficits following brain injury and their impact on psychosocial adjustment. *Cognitive Rehabilitation 1,* 4-7.

Russell, E. W.; Neuringer, C.; and Goldstein, G. 1970. *Assessment of Brain Damage: A Neuropsychological Key Approach.* New York: John Wiley and Sons.

Russell, W. R. 1971. *The Traumatic Amnesias.* London: Oxford University Press.

Rutter, M. 1981. Psychological sequelae of brain damage in children. *American Journal of Psychiatry 138(12),* 1533-1544.

Rutter, M.; Chadwick, O.; Shaffer, D.; and Brown, G. 1980. A prospective study of children with head injuries, I: Design and methods. *Psychological Medicine 11,* 49-61.

Sackheim, H. A.; Greenberg, M. S.; Weiman, A. L.; Gur, R. C.; Hungerbuhler, J. P.; and Geschwind, N. 1982. Hemispheric asymmetry in the expression of positive and negative emotions. *Archives of Neurology 39,* 210-218.

Sarno, M. T. 1976. The status of research in recovery from aphasia. In Y. Lebrun and R. Hoops, eds., *Recovery in Aphasics.* Amsterdam: Swets and Zeitlinger.

Schacter, D. L., and Crovitz, H. F. 1977. Memory function after closed head injury: A review of the quantitative research. *Cortex 13,* 150-176.

Schacter, S., and Singer, T. E. 1962. Cognitive, social, and physiological determinants of emotional state. *Psychological Review 69,* 379-397.

Schilder, P. 1934. Psychic disturbances after head injuries. *American Journal of Psychiatry 91,* 155-188.

Shaffer, D.; Chadwick, O.; and Rutter, M. 1975. Psychiatric outcome of localized head injury in children. In CIBA Foundation, *Outcome of Severe Damage to the Nervous System.* New York: Elsevier-North Holland Publishing Co.

Simon, H. A. 1967. Motivation and emotional controls of cognition. *Psychological Review 74,* 29-39.

Sullivan, H. S. 1933. *The Interpersonal Theory of Psychiatry.* New York: W. W. Norton and Co.

Taylor, E. M. 1959. *Psychological Appraisal of Children with Cerebral Defects.* Cambridge, Mass.: Harvard University Press.

Timbergen, N. 1953. *Social Behavior in Animals.* London: Methuen.

Tornatore, F. L.; Lee, D.; and Sramek, J. J. (1981). Psychotic exacerbation with haloperidol. *Drug Intelligence and Clinical Pharmacy 15,* 209-213.

Ullmann, L. P., and Krasner, L. 1967. The psychological model. In T. Millon, ed., *Theories of Psychopathology.* Philadelphia: W. B. Saunders Co.

Valenstein, E., and Heilman, K. M. 1979. Emotional disorders resulting from lesions of the central nervous system. In K. M. Heilman and E. Valenstein, eds., *Clinical Neuropsychology.* New York: Oxford University Press.

Van Zomeren, A. H. 1981. *Reaction Time and Attention After Closed Head Injury.* Amsterdam: Swets and Zeitlinger.

Van Zomeren, A. H., and Deelman, B. G. 1978. Long-term recovery of visual reaction time after closed head injury. *Journal of Neurology, Neurosurgery, and Psychiatry 41,* 452-457.

Voth, H., and Orth, M. H. 1973. *Psychotherapy and the Role of the Environment.* New York: Behavioral Publications.

Walker, A. E. 1972. Long-term evaluation of the social and family adjustment to head injuries. *Scandinavian Journal of Rehabilitative Medicine 4,* 5–8.

Wechsler, D. 1945. *Manual for the Wechsler Memory Scale, Form I.* New York: Psychological Corporation.

———. 1955. *Manual – Wechsler Adult Intelligence Scale.* New York: Psychological Corporation.

———. 1981. *Wechsler Adult Intelligence Scale – Revised Form Manual.* New York: Psychological Corporation.

Weddell, R.; Oddy, M.; and Jenkins, D. 1980. Social adjustment after rehabilitation: A two-year follow-up of patients with severe head injury. *Psychological Medicine 10,* 257–263.

Weinberg, J.; Diller, L.; Gordon, W.; Gerstman, L.; Lieberman, A.; Lakin, P.; Hodges, G.; and Izrachi, O. 1977. Visual scanning training effect on reading-related tasks in acquired right brain damage. *Archives of Physical Medicine and Rehabilitation 58,* 479–486.

Weinberg, J.; Piasetsky, E.; Diller, L.; and Gordon, W. 1982. Treating perceptual organizational deficits in non-neglecting RBD stroke patients. *Journal of Clinical Neuropsychology 4,* 59–75.

Weinstein, E. A., and Kahn, R. L. 1955. *Denial of Illness.* Springfield, Ill.: Charles C Thomas Publishing Co.

Weinstein, E. A., and Keller, N. A. 1963. Linguistic patterns of misnaming in brain injury. *Neuropsychologia 1,* 79–90.

Weinstein, E. A.; Marvin, S. L.; and Keller, N. A. 1962. Amnesia as a language pattern. *Archives of General Psychiatry 6,* 259–270.

Wilson, B. A., and Moffat, N. 1984. *Clinical Management of Memory Problems.* London: Aspen Publications.

Woods, B. T. 1980. The restrictive effects of right hemisphere lesions. *Neuropsychologia 18,* 65–70.

Yalom, I. D. 1970. *The Theory and Practice of Group Psychotherapy.* New York: Basic Books.

Zangwill, O. L. 1947. Psychological aspects of rehabilitation in cases of brain injury. *British Journal of Psychology 37,* 60–69.

Author Index

Page numbers in italics indicate chapter author

Abraham, J., 172
Achenbach, T. M., 44, 165
Adams, J. H., xix, 1, 165, 168
Adams, K. M., 170
Anthony, W. A., 140, 165
Arana, G., 167
Avezaat, C., 168

Bach, S. R., 84, 86, 165
Baker, G., 99, 118, 165
Baldessarini, R., 167
Barr, A. J., 124, 165
Barth, J. T., 172
Bear, D. M., 13, 33, 165, 167
Benowitz, L., 167
Benson, D. F., 18, 19, 29, 42, 165, 166
Benton, A. L., xix, 169
Ben-Yishay, Y., 6, 13, 52, 55, 64, 98, 118, 165–166, 167
Blumer, D., 29, 166
Boll, T. J., 172
Boller, F., 170
Bond, M. R., 9, 16, 47, 69, 93, 96, 99, 102, 120, 126, 130, 135, 166, 172
Braakman, R., 120, 166, 168
Brooks, D. N., 16, 65, 96, 102, 120, 126, 166, 170
Brown, G., 34, 43, 44, 166, 173
Bruckner, F. E., 9, 47, 48, 96, 99, 131, 166
Buss, A. H., 47, 166
Butters, N., 9, 166

Caton, W., 168
Caveness, W. F., 167

Chadwick, O., 43, 68, 166, 173
Chelune, G. J., 168
Crisco, J. J., 169
Crovitz, H. F., 8, 173
Cummings, N. A., 118, 166
Curtis, B. A., 43, 166

Darley, F. L., 52, 55, 167
David, C., 170
Davison, L., 122, 172
Dean, P., 70, 167
Deelman, B. G., 5, 173
Dennerll, R. D., 15, 69, 167
Dikmen, S., 16, 35, 167, 170
Diller, L., 13, 52, 55, 63, 98, 165–166, 167, 174
Dimascio, A., 170
Doyle, D., xix, 168
Dresser, A. C., 11, 48, 167

Eccles, J. C., 3, 167
Edelbrock, C. S., 44, 165

Fahy, T. J., 96, 167
Ferguson, S. M., 8, 40, 167
Fingers, S., 52, 167
Finklestein, S., 41, 167
Flavell, J. H., 3, 167
Fordyce, D. J., *1,* 13, *18,* 36, 93, *96,* 99, 102, 116, *119,* 120, 122, 130, 167, 172, 173
Freedman, A. M., 30, 40, 41, 167
Freud, S., 30, 47, 167
Fuster, J. M., 6, 42, 168

Author Index

Gainotti, G., 37, 41, 168
Galanter, E., 170
Galbraith, S., 168
Gans, J. S., 135, 168
Gasparrini, B., 10, 52, 65, 168
Gazzaniga, M. S., 63, 168
Gelpke, G. J., 166
Gennarelli, T. A., 1, 13, 171
Gerstman, L., 165, 166, 174
Geschwind, N., 19, 168, 173
Gianutsos, J., 10, 52, 65, 168
Gianutsos, R., 10, 52, 65, 168
Gilchrist, E., 47, 99, 119, 168
Gill, M. M., 30, 171
Giordani, B., 172
Goldstein, G., 173
Goldstein, K., 1, 29, 30, 33, 34, 35, 51, 52, 53, 55, 83, 90, 98, 99, 102, 118, 134, 168
Gonzalez, S., 167
Goodkin, R., 167
Goodnight, J. H., 165
Gordon, W. A., 13, 165, 166, 167, 174
Graham, D. I., xix, 9, 33, 168
Grant, H., 168
Grant, I., 170
Green, P. E., 124, 168
Greenberg, M. S., 173
Griffith, E., 172
Gronwall, D., 10, 102, 168
Grossman, R. G., xix, 34, 35, 41, 69, 99, 169
Groswasser, Z., 170
Gur, R. C., 173

Habbema, J.D.F., 166
Halstead, W. C., 12, 168
Hawryluk, G., 172
Heaton, R. K., 15, 131, 168, 170, 171
Heiden, J., 168
Heilman, K. M., 13, 33, 37, 168, 173
Helwig, J. T., 165
Hodges, G., 174
Hogarty, G. E., 124, 168
Humphrey, M., 171
Hungerbuhler, J. P., 173

Irving, M. H., 167
Izrachi, O., 174

Jackson, H., 53
Jacobson, S., 166

Jane, J. A., 172
Jansen, M. A., 140, 165
Jenkins, D., 174
Jennett, B., 46, 120, 168
Johnston, C., 49, 170
Jung, C. G., 30, 84, 169

Kahn, R. L., 8, 12, 13, 21, 36, 174
Kaplan, E. F., 165
Kaplan, H. I., 167
Katz, M. M., 124, 168
Keller, N. A., 19, 21, 174
Kelly, P. J., 169
Kertesz, A., 52, 55, 169
Killam, K. F., 170
Kim, Y., 170
Kinsbourne, M., 63, 169
Kozol, H. L., 33, 169
Krasner, L., 68, 173
Kuffler, S. W., 3, 169
Kun, L. E., 44, 169
Kurze, T., 168

Labaw, W., 37, 169
Lackner, J. R., 19, 26, 169
Lakin, P., 166, 174
Lazarus, R. S., 31, 169
Lee, D., 173
Leftoff, S., 8, 40, 169
Lehman, A. W., 171
Lehman, R.A.W., 168
Levin, D. P., 172
Levin, H. S., xix, 1, 2, 3, 8, 11, 12, 18, 19, 21, 34, 35, 41, 52, 69, 99, 102, 169
Levine, D., 167
Lewin, W. N., 120, 169
Lezak, M. D., 46, 100, 114, 169
Liberman, A., 174
Lin, Y., 167
Lindsley, D. B., 30, 169
Lipper, S., 38, 169
Lipsitz, N., 172
Lipton, M. A., 38, 170
Lishman, W. A., 34, 35, 39, 41, 170
Lorenz, K., 30, 170
Luria, A. R., 3, 6, 19, 32, 51, 54, 55, 98, 118, 170, 171

Maas, A.I.P., 166, 168
Maeser, M. A., 165
Mandleberg, I. A., 102, 166, 170
Marcus, E. M., 166

Author Index

Marin, O. S., 20, 170
Marshall, T. F., 169
Martin, J. R., 172
Mash, E. J., 49, 170
McCabe, P., 52, 55, 169
McGuinness, D., 32, 171
McLean, A., 33, 170
McNeel, M. L., 167
McSweeny, A. R., 20, 170
Meirowsky, A. M., 167
Mendelson, L., 170
Meyers, C. A., 169
Millac, P., 167
Miller, E., 31, 52, 65, 170
Miller, G. A., 170
Miller, J. D., 172
Minderhoud, J. M., 166, 168
Mintz, N., 170
Moffat, N., 65, 174
Morgan, S. F., 16, 167
Morrow, L., 37, 170
Moya, K., 167
Mulhern, R. K., 169

Najenson, T., 96, 170, 172
Naydin, V. L., 170
Neuringer, C., 173
Newcombe, F., 3, 54, 170
Newnan, O. S., 15, 171
Nicholls, J. G., 3, 169

Oddy, M., 12, 14, 96, 171, 174
Ommaya, A. K., 1, 13, 171
Orr, W. C., 172
Orth, M. H., 67, 68, 173

Parsons, O. A., 10, 20, 120, 171, 172
Pendleton, M. T., 131, 168
Pepping, M., *119,* 172
Pickard, J., 168
Poeck, K., 171
Pribram, K. H., 3, 8, 30, 31, 32, 40, 170, 171, 172
Prigatano, G. P., *1,* 2, 8, 10, 11, 13, 16, *18,* 20, *29,* 30, 35, 36, 41, 44, *51,* 52, 61, 64, *67, 96,* 102, 116, *119,* 120, 122, 130, *134,* 167, 171-172

Randle, A.P.H., 9, 47, 48, 96, 99, 131, 166
Ratcliff, G., 3, 170
Rattok, J., 166

Rayport, M., 167
Reitan, R. M., 35, 41, 122, 167, 172
Rimel, R. W., 1, 16, 172
Roberts, A. H., 81, 169, 172
Rochester, S. R., 23, 172
Rodin, E. A., 167
Romano, M. D., 100, 172
Rose, J. E., 169
Rosenbaum, M., 64, 172
Rosenthal, M., 51, 172
Ross, B., 166
Roueche, J. R., 13, *18, 119,* 167, 172, 173
Russell, E. W., 122, 173
Russell, W. R., xix, 8, 173
Rutter, M., 43, 44, 49, 68, 173

Sackheim, H. A., 33, 173
Sadock, B. J., 167
Saffran, E. M., 170
Sall, P., 165
Sampson, H., 10, 102, 168
Sarno, M. T., 52, 55, 173
Sarwar, M., 169
Satz, P., 10, 52, 65, 168
Schacter, D. L., 8, 173
Schacter, S., 31, 173
Schechter, I., 170
Schilder, P., 33, 39, 173
Schwartz, M. F., 170
Schwartz, M. L., 167
Shaffer, D., 44, 68, 166, 173
Silver, S., 166
Simon, G. A., 167
Simon, H. A., 3, 30, 31, 42, 173
Singer, T. E., 31, 173
Small, R., 168
Sramek, J. J., 173
Stahl, M. L., 172
Staz, P., 168
Stoll, A., 167
Stuss, D. T., 165
Sullivan, H. S., 30, 173

Taylor, E. M., 43, 173
Teasdale, G., 168, 169
Temkin, N. R., 170
Thomas, L., 166
Thurston, S., 172
Timbergen, N., 30, 173
Timms, R. M., 170
Tornatore, F. L., 38, 173

Traub, M., 166
Tsvetkova, L. W., 170
Tuchman, M. M., 38, 169

Ullmann, L. P., 68, 173
Uttley, D., 171

Valenstein, E., 173
Van Zomeren, A. H., 5, 173
Vecht, F., 168
Vinarskava, E. N., 170
Voth, H., 67, 68, 173
Vrtunski, K., 170

Walker, A. E., 48, 96, 174
Wechsler, D., 174
Weddell, R., 9, 14, 16, 34, 47, 48, 49, 96, 119, 131, 174
Weiman, A. L., 173
Weinberg, J., 52, 63, 65, 167, 174

Weinstein, E. A., 8, 12, 13, 19, 21, 23, 27, 36, 174
Weir, W. S., 165
Weiss, G. H., 167
Weschler, D., 122
Wienecke, R., 67
Wilkinson, M., 47, 99, 119, 168
Wilson, B. A., 65, 174
Woo, E., 167
Wood, B. C., *119,* 172
Woods, B. T., 43, 174
Wright, E., 172
Wrightson, P., 168
Wyler, A. R., 170

Yalom, I. D., 82, 174

Zangwill, O. L., 51, 52, 53, 54, 55, 59, 63, 98, 116, 118, 174
Zeiner, H. K., 44, *119,* 172

Subject Index

Abstract attitude, impairment of, 52–53, 83, 90
Abstraction, problems of, 102
Acceptance, 67, 100, 104–106, 132, 140–141
Affective disturbances, 29, 41; and nonaphasic linguistic difficulty, 21
Allesthesia, 13
Amnesia, 8, 13, 35
Amnestic disturbances, 5, 90; and use of third person in speech, 23
Amotivational states, 34, 41–43
Amphetamines, 38
Amygdala: damage to, 39; role of, in feeling states, 32
Analogies, 73
Anomia, 5, 11
Anosodiaphoria, 13
Anosognosia, 13. See also Denial-of-illness syndrome
Anticholinergics, 54
Anxiety, 34–36, 90–91; and degree of brain damage, 35
Aphasia, 11, 18, 55, 102; definition of, 18; forms of, 19
Arousal, alteration of: after brain injury, 31; with right-hemisphere injury, 38
Arousal-orienting system, 13
Arteriovenous malformation (AVM), 60–61, 76
Artistic expression, 83
Attention, 65, 102; disorders of, 4, 5–6; alteration of: after brain injury, 31; with right-hemisphere injury, 38

Average Impairment Rating, 15, 102, 120, 122, 126, 127, 131
Awareness, 67, 100, 132
Awareness training, 103–106

Basal ganglia: ischemic damage to, and craniocerebral trauma, 9; role of, in motivation, 32
Behavioral problems, after brain injury, 68–69
Behavior modification, 72, 73. See also Cognitive remediation
Body image, 14, 46, 82
Brain: areas of, at risk in severe head injury, 1–2, 13; ischemic damage to, xix, 9; reorganization of, after injury, 53–54
— function: alterations in, after trauma, xix; "deinhibition" of, 54; plasticity of, 63
— injury: consequences of, 97; psychosocial consequences of, 46–49; related to psychiatric or behavioral disorders, 34
Brain stem, 1, 13; disturbances in, 31–32; injuries to, 10
Broca's aphasia, 19, 35

Catastrophic reaction, 34–36, 66, 79, 81, 107, 108, 116; and denial, 37; development of, 36
Cerebellum, ischemic damage to, 9
Cerebral cortex, ischemic damage to, 9
Child Behavioral Checklist, 43–44
Children, brain-injured: personality

179

Children, brain-injured (*continued*)
disturbances in, 43-44; psychiatric sequelae in, 68
Cognition: definition of, 3, 51; disordered, 40
Cognitive confusion, 33, 34, 56; and feeling states, 84; reduction of, 56
Cognitive deficits, 90, 102; definition of, 51; remediation of, 104
Cognitive dysfunction, 42; classification of, 16; common psychosocial outcomes of, 4-12; definition of, 3-4; patient's awareness of, 13; psychosocial outcomes of, 3-5; related to area of injury, 1; residual, predictors of, 1; treatment of, 16-17
Cognitive functions: after brain injury, xix, 1; interconnectedness of, 98
Cognitive group therapy, 59, 72, 104-106, 162; clinical example of, 106-107
Cognitive rehabilitation. *See* Cognitive remediation
Cognitive remediation, xix, xx, 32, 45, 51, 99, 116, 160; clinical example of, 110-112; clinical perspective, 56-64; historical perspective, 52-56; milieu approach to, 64; modules, 64; program, 102-104; rationale for, 98; research perspective, 64-66; steps in, 56-57; transfer or generalization effects of, 63-64
Cognitive retraining. *See* Cognitive remediation
Communication, disorders of, 5, 11-12
Compensation, 53-54, 57, 116
Compensation training, 10, 55, 57-61, 63-66, 103, 160
Competency, rating of, 13-14. *See also* Patient competency rating
Concentration, disorders of, 4, 5-6
Concrete thinking, 104
Confabulation, 24-25
Confusional state, 13
Coping, postinjury strategies of, 139-140

Denial, 13, 14
Denial-of-illness syndrome, 8, 13, 34, 36-38, 82, 100
Dependency, 15, 16, 46, 49
Depression, after brain injury, 15, 34, 41-43, 90-91
Dextroamphetamine, 38

"Disordered condition," 34
Distractibility, 6, 42
Divorce, adjustment of brain-injured person to, 88-89
Dopamine, 38
Drawings, by brain-injured patients, *facing 84, facing 85,* 85-87
Duncan Multiple-Range Test, 140

Electroconvulsive therapy (ECT), 92
Emotion: and cognition, 3; definition of, 31; problems of, after brain injury, xix, 33, 81
Employment, 46; after brain injury, 116-117, 119; and milieu training, 64-65; variables predicting, 15-16. *See also* Work

Family of brain-injured person: as cause of psychiatric disturbance in brain-injured child, 44, 68; education of, 92-94; intervention with, 69, 100; involvement of, in neuropsychological rehabilitation, 4, 63; problems of, 82; psychotherapy with, 92-94, 100; rating of patient's competence by, 13-14; reactions of, to brain-injured person, 81, 93-94, 135, 153-154; support for, xx. *See also* Spouse of brain-injured person
Family counseling, 114
Fatigability, 4, 5, 33
Feelings, 30-31; dealing with, in group therapy, 79-80, 107-108; perception and interpretation, disturbances in, after brain injury, 31-32
Finger Tapping Test, 122
Follow-up interview, 124, 125
Friendships, loss of, 49
Frontal gyrus, left, lesions of, 19
Frontal lobe: anterior, 1; dysfunction of, 8, 42; injury to, 89, 116-117
"Frontal lobe personality syndrome," 29
Frontal poles, 13

Goal-directed activities, disorders of, 4, 6-7
God, 84
Group cognitive retraining, 161-162. *See also* Cognitive remediation
Group psychotherapy. *See* Psychotherapy, group

Subject Index

Haloperidol, 38–39
Halstead Category Test, 12, 20
Halstead-Reitan Test Battery, 10, 20, 122; mean scores of NRP patients on, 137
Health maintenance organizations (HMOs), 118
Hemi-akinesia, 13
Hemi-inattention, 13
Hemispatial neglect, 13
Hemispheres. See Left hemisphere; Right hemisphere
Hippocampus, ischemic damage to, and craniocerebral trauma, 9
Hostility, in family of brain-injured person, 93
Hyperactivity, 44
Hypothalamus: lateral region, role of, in motivation, 32; role of, in feeling states, 32

Impulsivity, xix, 2, 4, 33, 34–35, 104; in children, 44
Inattention, 104
Information-processing, 102, 110; deficits in, 13; disorders of speed of, 5, 10–11; and employability, 15
Initiation, disorders of, 4, 6–7
Insurance carriers, role of, in rehabilitation program, 158, 159
Interpersonal relationships, changes in, after brain injury, 47–49
Irritability, xix, 16, 33

Judgment: disorders of, 4, 7–8; impaired, after brain injury, xix, 2

Katz-R Adjustment Scale, 11, 12, 20–21, 35, 122, 127, 140; scores of NRP patients and controls on, 129

Language disturbances, 19; nonaphasic, 11–12, 18–28, 104. See also Peculiar phraseology
Language therapy, 161
Learning, disorders of, 4–5, 8–10, 102
Left hemisphere: and catastrophic reaction, 35; injury to, 11, 18, 86
— lesions: and denial-of-illness syndrome, 37–38; and language disturbances, 18, 19

Memory: disorders of, 4–5, 8–10; problems of, after brain injury, xix, 2, 24–26, 48, 55, 102, 104; retraining of, 61–62, 65; short-term, 61
Milieu approach, 55, 64–65, 100, 113, 154, 163
Minnesota Multiphasic Personality Inventory (MMPI), 14
Motivation: and cognition, 3; definition of, 31; disturbances in, 32–33; problems of, after brain injury, xix, 81
Motor movement, speed of, 15
Motor planning, disorder in kinetics of, 6–7

Neuroleptics, 38
Neuropsychological rehabilitation: effectiveness of, 130–131; interdisciplinary approach to, 99–100; 114–115; practical considerations in, 153–154. See also Outcome of treatment; Presbyterian Hospital, Oklahoma City, Neuropsychological Rehabilitation Program of
Neuropyschological Rehabilitation Program (NRP). See Presbyterian Hospital, Oklahoma City, Neuropsychological Rehabilitation Program of
Neuropsychological testing. See Testing
Neuropsychology, 30

Occupational therapy, 161
"Ordered condition," 34
Outcome of treatment: determinants of, 135–136; failure, 138–139; initial evaluation of, 115–118; measures of, 117–118; predictors of, 138–139; psychosocial, 3–4, 46–49; social and neurological, 5; success, 132, 138, 140; variables influencing, 120. See also Presbyterian Hospital, Oklahoma City, Neuropsychological Rehabilitation Program of

Paranoia, 34, 38–40, 90, 91
Paranoid ideation, xix, 8, 24–25, 34, 38, 40, 82
Parents of brain-injured children, psychiatric illness in, 49
Patient competency rating: patient's form, 143–146; relative's form, 147–151

Peculiar phraseology, 12, 23–27
Perception, disorders of, 4, 7–8, 102
Perseveration, 4, 7
Personality: definition of, 30, 81; development of, 43; neuropsychological considerations of, 30–33
— change, 29, 49, 82; with brain lesions, 29; and employment, 16; and memory disturbance, 9
— disorders, 69; after brain injury, xix, 33–43; classification of, 44–46; and rehabilitation, 10
— disturbances, 49–50, 99, 107–108, 116; affective, 29; in brain-injured children, 43–44; over time, 93; treatment of, 16–17, 72
— premorbid, 111, 132; discussion of, 109; influence of, on postmorbid personality, 33–34; and paranoid ideation, 40; problems with, 107–108; and resistance to therapy, 91
— problems, 53, 55; characterological, 44–46, 74; long-term, 45; neuropsychologically based, 45–46, 74, 108–109; reactionary, 44–46, 74
Personality tests, 122–124; findings of, 127–128
Physical therapy, 160–161
Prefrontal lobe, injuries to, 6–7
Presbyterian Hospital, Oklahoma City, Neuropsychological Rehabilitation Program of, 102–114; cost-efficiency of, 117, 154; cost of, to patient, 158; daily schedule in, 155–156; effectiveness of, 130–132; evaluation of, 157–158; financial considerations in, 158–159; format of, 155–156; medical consultants in, 114; modification of, 134–142; outcome of, 119–133; philosophy of, 98–100, 155; problem areas addressed by, 152–153; purposes of, 152; rationale for, 98–100; referral of patients to, 158; Relatives' Group, 114, 163; revisions to, 152–163; services offered by, 154, 159–163; staff of, 114–115, 157–158; work trial following (*see* Work trial, following rehabilitation)
— patients: demographic and neurological characteristics of, 121, 136; selection of, 100–102; "successes" and "failures," 136–137; types of, considered appropriate, 154–155
Problem-solving, strategies of, 4, 102, 103
Psychiatric illness: after head injury, 68; premorbid, and failure in psychotherapy, 92
Psychomotor agitation, 34, 38–40
Psychotherapy: definition of, 67–68; for family members, 92–94; individual, 74–77; misperceptions of, 74, 75; predictable issues arising in, 88–92
— after brain injury, xix, xx, 44, 68, 99, 108, 161; effectiveness of, 67–68, 118; elements of, 71–74; goals of, 69–71; schema for conducting, 74; success of, 99
— group, 72, 74, 77–83, 107–110, 162; aims of, 79; conducting, 79–80; difficulties in, 80; selection of patients for, 78–79; topics discussed in, 80–82

Reasoning, impairment of, 32
Recovery, after brain injury: level of, possible, 116; model of stages of, 105
Relatives. *See* Family of brain-injured person; Spouse of brain-injured person
Resistance, 90, 100
Restlessness, 20, 38
Retraining: direct, 54, 63, 64, 66; perceptual, 65; psychomotor, 65–66. *See also* Cognitive remediation
Right hemisphere: infarct, 13
— lesions, 36; and denial-of-illness syndrome, 37–38; and language problems, 19
Russell-Neuringer Average Impairment Rating. *See* Average Impairment Rating

"Schizophreniform" psychosis, 39
Self-appraisal, after brain injury, 12–14, 16
Self-awareness: after brain injury, 48; problems of, 12
Self-confidence, 82
Self-esteem, reduced, 46
Self-perception, altered, 7–8
Sexual dysfunction, 82

Sexual feelings, of brain-injured person toward therapist, 90
Social competency, role of, in treatment success, 139–141
Social inappropriateness, 106, 111
Social isolation, 79, 82
Social withdrawal, 34, 41–43
Speech therapy, 161
Spouse of brain-injured person: psychiatric illness in, 49; psychotherapy for, 94. See also Family of brain-injured person
Staff of rehabilitation program: commitment of, 135; development of, 114–115; interdisciplinary relationships among, 114–115; meetings of, 113–114; rating of patient's competence by, 13–14; reactions of, to brain-injured patients, 94–95, 135; support for, xx
Substitution, 53–54
Substitution training, 63–66
Suicide, 91–92
Symbolism, in therapeutic process, 83–88

Tactual Performance Test, 122, 127
Talkativeness, 5, 11–12, 20–21, 27, 104
Tangentiality, 5, 6, 11–12, 21–23, 27, 104, 106
Temporal gyrus, superior left, lesions in, 19
Temporal lobe: anterior, 1; dysfunction of, 8, 34; injury to, 89–90, 116–117; left, 39; medial, lesions of, 39; role of, in feeling states, 32; role of, in visual discrimination, 40
Testing, after brain injury: 122; analysis of, 127–127; mean scores of NRP patients, 137–138; role of, in patient selection, 100–101; variables affecting, 122. See also names of specific tests
Thalamus, lesions in, and quasi-aphasic disturbances, 19–20

Therapy: independent supervised, 113; individual, 160–161. See also Electroconvulsive therapy; Family of brain-injured person, psychotherapy with; Language therapy; Occupational therapy; Physical therapy; Psychotherapy, group; Speech therapy
Third person, patients' referral to self in, 23, 26
Trail Making Test, 10, 26, 122
Transference, 90

Unemployment, 14–16. See also Employment

Verbal expansiveness, 11–12. See also Talkativeness
Videotape, use of, in therapy, 104–107
Violence, 39: in paranoid patient, 91
Vocational counseling, 163

WAIS-R, 122
WAIS-R Vocabulary, 20
Wechsler Adult Intelligence Scale (WAIS), 20, 122; Digit symbol subtest of, 15, 131, 138
Wechsler Memory Scale, 7, 122
Wechsler test scores: mean, of NRP patients, 137; of NRP patients and controls, 126–127, 129–130
Wernicke's aphasia, 19
Withdrawal, 82
Word fluency, reduced, 11
Work, 82; assessing ability to, 47; and cognitive and personality disturbance, 99; follow-up statistics on, 128–132; memory skills and, 9; return to, predictors of, 9, 48. See also Employment
Work history, 132
Work trial, following rehabilitation, 131, 134, 152, 156–157, 163

The Johns Hopkins University Press

Neuropsychological Rehabilitation after Brain Injury

This book was composed in Times Roman text and display type by Capitol Communication Systems, from a design by Chris L. Smith. It was printed on S. D. Warren's 50-lb. Sebago Eggshell Cream Offset paper and bound in Holliston's Roxite A by BookCrafters, Inc.